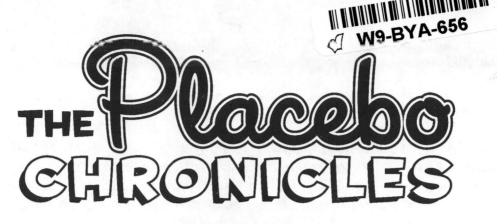

THE Placebo CHRONICLES

STRANGE but TRUE TALES from the DOCTOR'S LOUNGE

Douglas Farrago, M.D.

Illustrations by Gordon W. Marshall

Broadway Books
New York

BROADWAY

PRINTED IN THE UNITED STATES OF AMERICA

BROADWAY BOOKS and its logo, a letter B bisected on the diagonal, are trademarks of Random House, Inc.

Visit our website at www.broadwaybooks.com

First edition published 2005.

Book design by Gordon W. Marshall
Illustrated by Gordon W. Marshall

Cataloging-in-Publication Data is on file with the Library of Congress.

ISBN 0-7679-1949-1

10 9 8 7 6 5 4 3 2 1

I dedicate this book to my father, Allan G. Farrago.
Some of my fondest memories of you are when I made you smile.
You died too soon. I miss you, Pop.

CONTENTS

The Placebo Chronicles

INTRODUCTION

So, you think you know a little about a physician's life, huh?

You think just because you have seen a reality program showing an open-heart surgery or a baby being born that you know what physicians are going through? Well, I am here to tell you that you don't know diddly-squat. You are missing a big piece of the picture. Most physicians are on an emotional roller coaster that gets wilder each day. Did you know that forty percent of doctors feel burned out? Did you know that one in four doctors are on a medication for a psychiatric illness? **What does this mean to you?** A lot. ***With all this stress comes great stories!***

For the past two years *Placebo Journal* has been chronicling these stories. *Placebo Journal* is the only medical journal that makes its readers laugh and allows its contributors to vent their frustrations. Since most *Placebo Journal* readers and contributors are physicians, I feel that in some way the magazine has been providing a sort of therapy for this class of struggling professionals. Interestingly enough, however, as the number of humorous, gross, amazing, and interesting stories has grown, so have the numbers of laypeople who read them and love them. Sure, much of it may make their stomachs queasy, but like driving by an automobile accident, they can't look away. So I decided to open up the *Placebo Journal*'s story vault and publish *The Placebo Chronicles*. If you're a regular reader of *Placebo Journal*, you'll know my ulterior motive is to make some extra cash – Medicare and HMOs pay like crap nowadays.

You may be asking yourself, *"Is it okay for my doctor to laugh at his experiences, especially if they involve me?"* Not only is humor in medicine okay, but I think it is desperately needed. "Humor" and "medicine" may not seem like two words that go together naturally. But humor may be the only way for doctors to survive the increasing pressures of the medical profession. Our jobs as physicians can sometimes be dehumanizing and we may end up getting thick-skinned in order to survive emotionally. The problem is that physicians are, in fact, real people with real emotions. They are human like most of you *(there was a joke in there somewhere)*. Just because they took the Hippocratic Oath does not mean they promised to become RoboDocs. In fact, many of the same things that rattle your cage rattle theirs. You know that aunt who drives you crazy with her complaints about every ache and pain? *Remember where you always tell her to go?* To the doctor! *Well guess what?* She drives her doctor crazy, too.

The stories and opinions in *The Placebo Chronicles* come from physicians around the country. All of them are true. Forget *Marcus Welby MD, St. Elsewhere*, or even *ER*. ***You want reality?*** **Well, this book is it.** These are the stories that doctors tell each other while sitting in the doctors' lounge. These are the stories that doctors laugh together about at parties. These are the stories doctors commiserate about when considering switching careers.

more ☞

If you want philosophic advice, beautifully written prose, or thought-provoking concepts, then you need to look elsewhere.

If you want to laugh at the medical system as we know it and don't mind the offensive, you will love this book. We have stories from each stage of a doctor's life: medical student, resident, new doctor, and experienced doctor. We have stories about problematic patients: narcotic seekers and Munchausens. We will show you how doctors relate to HMOs, pharmaceutical companies, and much more. Plus, we have some pretty interesting X-rays that will beg the question, *"They put what in where?"*

Why the name? The Latin definition of a **"placebo"** is *"to give pleasure to."* Interestingly enough, just like a placebo pill, our journal sometimes produces a positive effect from something of very little substance (*as you will soon see*). Also, like the placebo, many times it does no good at all. Whether it's a placebo or not, I have found that editing this rag has been the best thing for my own mental health. *It is the psychotherapy that my HMO has repeatedly declined to cover.* **You see, I was burning out.** I slowly began to recognize the subtle signs. For example, I found myself buying lottery tickets to give to patients so that I could bribe them to go away and leave me alone. At other times I was pitting my male patients against each other in a cruel game of "bobbing for Viagra" using a bucket in my waiting room. **I needed help.** The answer I found was to share my stories, as deranged, unprofessional, and embarrassing as they might be, with other doctors. I realized that I was not alone out there. These shared experiences became the *Placebo Journal* and, now, *The Placebo Chronicles.*

Now let me be serious for a moment before you read on. We don't mean to denigrate the practice of medicine, our patients, or other physicians. We do mean to show the human side of the medical profession. Sure, we may mock or laugh at the mentally challenged, but what else are you going to say about hospital administrators? We don't print any stories in which a patient's care was compromised. Sometimes, however, you will find the stories cross the line of good, or even marginally acceptable, taste. They are crude, funny, and a telling commentary on the mental state of physicians today. **Live with it.** It's not like we write about doctors having sex with their patients. We are leaving that for the veterinarians.

Bottom line: There is no mission to change the world and this didn't take years of preparation, hundreds of focus groups, and tons of venture capital to get started. **The concept is simple; I want to make physicians laugh at themselves, their patients, and at medicine in general.** Without some sort of outlet such as humor, doctors run the very real risk of becoming desensitized to the human element in this profession. And without empathy, patient care standards suffer. Doctors who laugh regularly have a better shot at delivering good, compassionate care than those who are burned out, overwrought, and taking themselves too seriously.

Placebo Journal, and now *The Placebo Chronicles*, answer the command *"Doctor, heal thyself."* Now you get a chance to enter this secret world and laugh along with your doctor. *Just don't bust a gut doing it – he's overworked already.* ✚

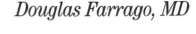
Douglas Farrago, MD

MEDICAL SCHOOL

INTRODUCTION

The long, grueling process of becoming a doctor begins with medical school. It's four years of hell after college. It was the hardest thing that I had to go through in my young life until, of course, residency, which was even worse (*you will read about that in the next chapter*).

Just getting into medical school is an incredible feat in itself, the first of many Darwinian trials an aspiring doctor faces. You need exceptionally high college grades, which isn't easy because competition grows stronger and stronger. As time goes on, the weakest students give up and the strongest students hang around, totally screwing up any type of testing curve. **The pressure to succeed is enormous.** I remember the shock of my first chemistry class in college. There were five hundred people in it and almost all of them, including me, wanted to go medical school. Only ten or twenty would succeed. No one would have predicted I would be one of those ten or twenty. **Not even me.**

In medical school, the whole competition process starts all over again. The testing is outrageously hard and the hours are ridiculously long. The first two years, the medical student actually has minimal patient contact since he or she is wrapped up doing the basics of science including biochemistry, neurology, chemistry, histology, etc. When the "clinical rotations" start in year three, the real fun (or horror) begins. Here is where the student spends months at a time seeing patients in such areas as internal medicine, surgery, emergency medicine, and obstetrics. Finally, young men and women who are tired of just the textbooks get a chance to try to treat live patients. This is a real eye-opener for them. This is when they start to see it all and feel it all. This is where they learn to develop their defenses against the gross, the sad, the disturbing, and the outrageous. I am not sure if having such thick skin is a good thing for doctors or not, but it is our basic survival mechanism to deal with these types of things. Seeing children die, arms that were severed, hearts splayed open, yellow patients, green patients, and blue patients are shocking, but a reality nonetheless. Any time taken to wallow in their own pity only takes time away from seeing other patients. The student buries his or her emotions to do his or her job and learns a valuable lesson: **Medicine is not pretty.**

I remember in my first anatomy class there was this sweet girl who was initially very bothered by the cadavers. The school had done all the right stuff to slowly introduce the new students to their "bodies." There were prayer sessions for those so inclined. There were warm-up periods so that people could acclimate to the cadaver. Still, people were squeamish, especially this one young woman. I didn't pay her too much attention because I had enough work to do on my own cadaver. I had totally forgotten about this student until halfway through the semester when I saw her walking by, whistling, with a sawed-off leg over her shoulder like a slab of meat. I thought to myself, *"Haven't we got a little sassy?"*

Now picture yourself as a medical student. See yourself trying to save a life all the while questioning whether you know what you are doing. You're nervous and exhausted. You're hungry and overworked. All you care about is sleep (and hoping you don't kill someone). As you become more and more disconnected from the real world, you fall more and more into the medical one. All you can remember are the basics of survival and those weird, gross or outrageous experiences that occurred during your dreamful "medical student" state. It is these patient encounters or stories, however, which you will remember forever. It is these stories you will collect like a hobby. They are ones you will never share with patients and only occasionally share with one another. They're not for the faint of heart but they are yours and yours only – *until now*. The following stories are ones that we have pried, bribed, or extorted from former medical students who have endured this torture. Their collection is now, for the first time, open for your perusal, but it comes at a cost. After reading them, you may become thick-skinned yourself and for that we have but one cure – **humor.** These doctors didn't laugh about their medical student experiences at the time, but trust us, they are laughing about it now. We hope you can do the same. ✚

ST▲GE꜔ of the PHYSI◠IA.J

I want to help people.
I want to make it through this hell.
I want to make it through this hell without killing someone.
I may have killed someone.
I want someone to help me.

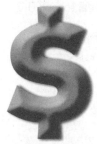

I want to make money.
I want to spend money.
I want to save money.
Where the hell is my money?
I need to make money.

I don't know anything.
There is too much to know.
I will never know all of this.
I don't need to know all of this.
I only need to know a little.
I don't care if I know anything.

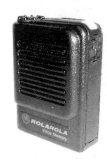

I want to be needed.
I love my white jacket.
I love the power of the pager.
I hate this f*cking pager.
I don't want to wear a stupid jacket.
I want to be left alone.

This patient has some interesting problems.
This patient has some real disease.
This patient needs to be hugged and loved.
This patient has a lot of nothing.
This patient has Sh*tty Life Syndrome.
This patient needs to leave; I need to be
    hugged and loved.✚

5

MEDICAL STUDENTS' REVENGE

Our OB-GYN rotation at a busy inner-city hospital was one of the most grueling of medical school. The residents were miserable and as all miserable residents do, they torture medical students for relief. One particularly sadistic senior resident was on call with us on Friday night, one of the busiest of the service. He would extract as much scut from us as possible and he was merciless in his criticism. Any procedure we would attempt was quickly taken over by this impatient resident. Since it was the last day of the rotation, I was eager to finish a call and never touch a speculum again. My medical student colleague, however, had only revenge on his mind.

At around 3 a.m., we were called to the ER to work up a morbidly obese patient with *"itching down there."* After our thorough history and cursory physical, we called the senior resident. In his usually abrupt manner, he dismissively listened to our presentation and proceeded into the room for the exam. The patient put her legs on the stirrups, but as with most morbidly obese patients, there was no hint of the vagina except the odor and converging folds of endless flesh. Even the sweat in between the rolls of cellulite gave an additional pungency to the aroma.

"I'm sorry I'm so fat, doctor," she kept repeating half sleepily. With much reluctance, we each held back a thigh so our fearless leader could plunge into the depths with his speculum for his examination. As our resident diligently probed flesh with his speculum, my medical student colleague looked up at me with a gleam in his eye and a wink . . .

Thwack!!

He had let go of his thigh and I instinctively did the same . . .

Thwack!!

I will never forget the seemingly headless senior resident flailing his arms trying to free himself from the deluge of flesh and odor that was delivered onto his bare cheeks. He was now cheek to cheek with our sleepy patient who barely reacted to the fracas. We quickly regained our composure and insincerely apologized to our resident, who tried his best to proceed with his exam. The rest of the evening just seemed to pass by effortlessly and our senior resident was much nicer to us for the remainder of the shift. ✚

ER STUFF

As a very green third-year medical student in Bellevue Hospital (NYC) emergency room, I spent much of the time wide-eyed and terrified. With its surreal mix of the heroic, overwhelming, and bizarre, Bellevue ER was a great place for memorable patients and events that have stayed fresh in my mind for years.

One shift I noticed a man on a stretcher having a grand mal seizure. This seemed to make absolutely no impression on the surrounding patients, or the staff for that matter. Just as I was really getting worried, a nurse strode past, said to the patient,

"Oh Jack, cut it out!" . . . and he did. ✚

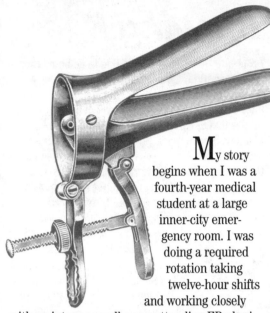

My story begins when I was a fourth-year medical student at a large inner-city emergency room. I was doing a required rotation taking twelve-hour shifts and working closely with an intern as well as an attending ER physician. I enjoyed the fast pace of the big city ER but did experience significant anxiety when a code was underway or an imminent or a major trauma was unfolding.

The attending wanted me to see patients, assess them, and formulate a plan. I went to see what seemed to be my 100th patient this shift. Ms. Greenjeans was a 76-year-old female who presented with nonspecific pelvic discomfort. She had the usual past medical history including diabetes, tobacco abuse, alcoholism and substance abuse, hypertension, renal insufficiency, etc. Her abdominal exam was unremarkable, but as we all know, "No abdominal exam is complete without a pelvic exam."

The forty-bed ER was nothing more than a large room separated by pull curtains that do provide visual privacy but do not provide much privacy in regard to conversation. In other words, the whole ER including patients, staff, etc., can hear every word I say to the patient.

Ms. Greenjeans was morbidly obese and **hard of hearing** so this pelvic exam would likely be difficult but, considering I had done two pelvic exams in my entire medical career (counting this one), I thought I could handle it.

Ms. Greenjeans was placed in the lithotomy position with lifting help from nursing (#1: because nurses are much stronger than doctors; #2: because all doctors have "a bad back"; #3: because this patient's legs resembled large, soft,

fleshy bags of cottage cheese). I reached for a speculum not realizing that they actually came in different sizes. By chance, I chose a medium-sized model and inserted it into the vagina. Unfortunately, due to the size of the patient, I could barely see the labia minora.

The ER nurse who was chaperoning my exam recommended a change in equipment. I looked up at the nurse with total confusion on my face as she handed me a jumbo-sized speculum resembling a small fishing vessel or salad tongs. I again inserted the instrument to get a better look into the vaginal vault. Words cannot describe the horror, surprise, and disgust as I watched several hundred maggots squirming to exit to the outside world. I jumped back suddenly, nearly falling on my butt. *"This could not be happening? Why me?"* I quickly ran over to my attending to tell him the news; he casually walked over to the business end of the exam table and confirmed my diagnosis.

"Yeah, those are MAGGOTS." He then informed me that I should tell the patient her diagnosis and then proceed with cleaning them out of there. Sounded like a plan, but, *why me, why here, and why now?* I stood up at the head of the exam table and in my best doctor voice I said, *"Ms. Greenjeans, you've got maggots in your vagina."* Suddenly the busy ER seemed so still, so quiet. I was sure everyone in the department could hear my every word. Ms. Greenjeans looked at me with a confused look on her face. She then yelled at the top of her lungs . . .

MAGNETS
HOW THE HELL DID MAGNETS GET IN THERE?

+

7

Talk About Blowing It

He was a passive guy and very laid back. When I saw him on the gurney I was surprised how calm he was. The ER physician had called earlier in the afternoon and stated that Frank was back because of his nausea and vomiting. He had a history of multiple admissions for gastroparesis from his diabetes. He truly had the latter disease and was insulin dependent. The gastroparesis was in question and previous testing never proved it. He was in his forties and had an obvious history of polysubstance abuse as well. He loved to smoke and drink and failed detox on many occasions. He also had chronic back problems, as well as the abdominal pain he claimed to have from his gastroparesis. His primary physician was tortured by him because she couldn't shed him from her practice. She had him on 60 mg of OxyContin three times a day and held him to a narcotic agreement/contract. He never overtly broke the contract, but when he would run out of his narcotic medication early he would coincidentally have severe nausea and vomiting and abdominal pain. Subsequently he would go to the ER for admission to cover those days he didn't have the medication he needed at home. Since dehydration can make diabetes lethal, it would be inappropriate to just ignore his demands and send him on his merry way. Even though no one ever saw him vomit in the ER, there was no one who would question Frank and chance the possibility of malpractice.

I knew Frank was a fraud and told him right away that I wouldn't give him any more medication to go home with when I discharged him. *He didn't bite.* I was expecting a fight but he just nodded quietly. He then rattled off the combination of antiemetics and narcotics he needed intravenously while he was an inpatient. It made the admission pretty easy and I put him in the hospital in about 10 minutes. By the second day of his admission, I had taken him off all his IV drugs and put him back on regular oral pain medication. Once again, no complaints. In fact, he was as nice as pie. Since I had never met Frank before, I was amazed at how easy admission was going and started to second guess the accusations about him.

THOSE DARN NARC SEEKERS

I told him that he should be able to go home the next day and he agreed wholeheartedly.

The next morning I was seeing a patient on the floor below Frank when I received a page by the nurses taking care of him. Since I was coming up in about five minutes, I didn't answer, figuring I would see the nurses personally. When I opened the stairwell door to enter Frank's floor I saw a huge commotion. About four nurses were buzzing around his room and two were frantic by the phone waiting for my call. Then I noticed that security personnel were mingling around as well. *This is not good*, I thought.

It seemed poor old Frank wasn't enjoying himself as much as he would have liked to. He was getting his normal dose of OxyContin as he would at home, but I guess there was more fun to be had. The morning nurse had walked into the room to find our friend in the corner snorting some "home" OxyContin that he snuck in with him. Initially he dumped it on the floor and spread it around as much as he could. Too late. The nurse confronted him and he confessed. They are tough birds who don't take no for an answer easily.

Never underestimate the stupidity of some people. Frank was being discharged that morning and he knew it. All he had to do was wait an hour and he could have gone home and had a party with his medication. No one would have known, and his charade would have continued indefinitely. Instead, Frank showed his impatience and blew it (literally). When I confronted Frank myself, I found a different man. He wasn't so nice anymore. He yelled at me. He cursed me out. He was ready to fight. As if in some way I was the bad guy, Frank put on a borderline personality show.

I finally ended our conversation by giving him two choices: discharge to home or detox. He chose to go to detox but left soon thereafter. Frank was discharged by his primary physician for lying about his drug use. I have a funny feeling that I will see Frank again on our "unassigned" service. My heart tells me that he won't stop his narcotic habit either.

My recommendation to readers of this encounter is to be a little leery of gastroparesis that sounds suspicious. It is a perfect alibi to get some pain meds for a joy ride. ✚

SMUDGE

This interesting diddy begins when I was a second-year resident at a large metropolitan teaching hospital. I was on-call one weekend during my Medicine Service rotation and hating life. A typical night on-call would involve somewhere in the neighborhood of four to eight admissions, a couple of ER blocks, and a whole lotta phone calls. My intern *(I love how attendings and senior residents refer to their students and interns or residents as "mine." It reminds me of slaves and indentured servants – which they are)* and I were called down to the ER for a patient with a deep venous thrombosis. We figured that this patient would take us about 8.5 minutes *(if we took our time)* to admit into the hospital as he had no other major medical problems. More importantly, my intern was "seasoned." This means that it was close to the end of the intern/resident cycle and he had seen this particular problem several times in the past year. He could therefore manage this almost completely on his own. This also meant that I could go get a cup of coffee while he did the whole damn thing and just about the time when he was done (maybe 8 minutes and 20 seconds along), I would appear and give a sound bite such as *"Looks like we need to get you in the big house and get this straightened out,"* or *"This looks like it's bad and needs fixin'."* Then I would review the intern's orders and drink more coffee. The teaching pearls for the case would come later while we reviewed the humorous or disgusting parts of the case.

I knew my intern was just about done with the admission when from across the ER I saw him move away from the patient and wave *(I was a trained medical observer you know)*. I quickly walked over to the patient's bedside and looked at his grossly swollen, red leg and proclaimed in my best authoritarian tone, *"This looks like the one! Let's get you upstairs and get to work."*

I then went to place the bed sheet back over his leg and something caught my eye.

Something was not right.

I had this strange feeling of a presence.

Something moved!

It turns out that this patient was the proprietor of a gay men's bar on the south side of town. He admitted to multiple sex partners in the recent past. As I focused on his groin, I could see what appeared to be a dirt smudge. A dirt smudge was not uncommon to see but a dirt smudge that was mobile was not an everyday occurrence. I moved in a little closer *(or was it farther away)* and saw a large gray and brown mass of small critters doing a line dance on his groin. I quickly turned to John *(my intern)* and asked him to take a closer look. I asked him to do it because there was no way in hell that I was going to. We both began to itch and feel the heebie-jeebies as the millions of critters switched from the line dance to the conga (dah, dah, dah, dah, dah, DAH!). What we had here was a good old-fashioned case of pubis pediculosis. That's crabs to you and me and it ain't the kind you eat.

I did what all experienced senior residents do. I got the hell out of there, but not before torturing the intern by making him get a painfully detailed sexual history including all STDs, previous partners, insect infestations, and the like. Sure he balked. Sure he was not motivated. It didn't matter because I was the boss and told him in no uncertain terms, *"Get right to it so I can get to sleep – and no nitpicking."*

Sometimes it's good to be the boss.

The lessons here were simple. Call always sucks. Always make sure your intern does a proper and full exam *(less you have to do)*.

And lastly . . . a smudge that moves is pretty damn gross, even if you are a physician. ✚

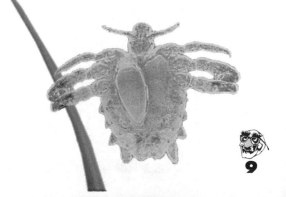

The title of
this image is

THE BIG ONE

Need we say more?

And ask yourself, "Is it a male or female?"

Will an X-Ray tell?

Right: Monster Vibrator in Colon

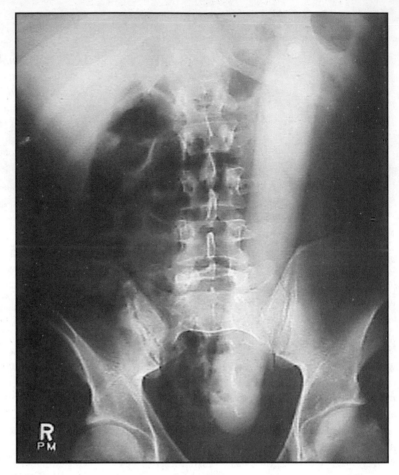

10

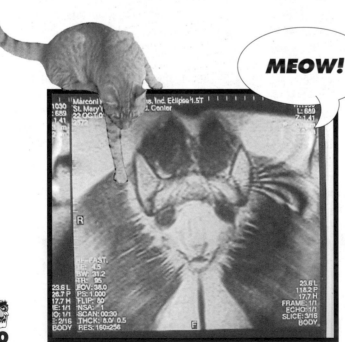

MEOW!

"**Here Kitty, Kitty...**"

You never know what will show up on an MRI scan . . .

"MEOW"

X-Ray Files

If we show you ours, will you show us yours?

You're seeing it all now . . .

"Rectal foreign bodies are a dime a dozen. Try to figure out what these are!"

ANSWER:
Scrotal Piercings. *A real Lord of the Rings!!*

A SALUTE TO
THE BARN

My first med school rotation was in surgery. I was assigned to a large teaching hospital in inner-city Philadelphia, the city of brotherly love. Like all new third-year students I was terrified. Upper classmen were always quick to tell their horror stories about particular rotations and this rotation was not one for the weak hearted. I did not have a whole lot of interest in surgery, I just got stuck with a tough rotation. Rounds began the first Monday of the rotation at 5 a.m. Patients were rounded on, with notes on the chart by 6 a.m. so that you could round again with the attending. After rounds (which lasted until about 9 a.m.)

it was off to the OR to become a human clamp/drain/suture holder while being pimped about anatomical triangles, triads, and trivia.

After lunch you would round again and await the ER and consult pages that steadily streamed in. *Good Times!* The house staff on the general surgery service consisted of the chief resident (slave driving, pimping, coffee drinking machine), several second-, third-, and fourth-year surgery residents, several interns, and a tribe of third- and fourth-year students.

We got a call from a general medical ward from the charge nurse telling us to get up to the floor stat to see this elderly lady with a large red mass protruding from her anus. My mind started to race, what the hell could it be?

I knew I had to think fast because the pimping would begin on the elevator up to the floor.

Cancer? Foreign body? Gerbil?

We reached the floor in a matter of moments. The patient's room was a large common room with six beds in it. The room was affectionately known as "The Barn," I guess due to the arrangement of the beds in stall-like fashion.

All of the patients in "The Barn" were demented, chronically ill, and smelled of urine and feces (just like the medical students).

There was music softly playing from a clock radio on the windowsill. I found out later in my career that this is standard operating procedure. The patients all were talking to themselves and seemed quite content. Mrs. Jones was our new patient. She was a 90-year-old demented black female. The chief resident gathered the house staff around her bed, and with great authority pulled back the sheets to reveal a large red mass protruding from the patient's anus! *Holy shit!* I thought.

What the hell is it?

(to my self of course . . . so I wouldn't be pimped). The chief resident and all of the surgical residents looked at one another and smiled. The interns looked at one another and grinned (like they knew what it was – but they didn't) and the students all looked at one another nervously.

The chief grabbed a latex glove and snapped it on his hand and with great manual dexterity took his index and middle fingers and stuffed the red mass back up this lady's anus. He then proclaimed,

"It's a prolapsed rectum,"

. . . and then he quickly yelled *"Grab some gloves,"* and pointed his clean fingers at me (he didn't know my name). I was terrified but excited that I was the chosen one, yet I was not sure why he chose me. He withdrew his fingers and Mrs. Jones's rectum quickly squirted out again onto the sheets. The chief then bellowed,

"Stuff it back in like this,"

. . . and he proceeded to show me the proper technique using my fingers. So now my fingers are firmly up this 90-year-old demented lady's butt in the middle of The Barn. I thought,

Wow! this is REAL medicine.

The chief then quickly walked out of the room with the rest of the house staff in tow. He said *"We'll be right back, don't move your fingers."* I sat there in that room with my fingers in this lady's rectum listening to the soft music and the sound of demented folks talking to themselves.

This went on for about an hour before I realized that the surgical service was not coming back. Yes I'm an idiot. *Bastards!* I finally got the courage to withdraw my fingers, wash my hands, and return to the surgery department to check in with the guys. Needless to say, they were all pissing themselves laughing and giving me

THE TWO-FINGER SALUTE.

I hate surgery. ✚

MEDICAL SCHOOL MISHAPS

As a third-year medical student, I was performing the admission examination on a **a beautiful and well-endowed young woman** admitted for possible acute bacterial endocarditis.

With my fellow student watching, I auscultated her heart and upon hearing a significant systolic murmur, placed the heel of my hand on her left parasternal area.

She inquired as to what I was doing whereupon I thoughtlessly replied,

"I am feeling for a thrill."
✚

Why I'll NEVER forget

The summer of 1992 was the start of my third year of medical school and therefore the start of clinical rotations. You remember when you were so excited that you didn't have to sit in classes anymore, but you were also scared shitless that you actually might have to touch a patient. Or worse yet, you might have to touch a certain part of that patient. This, my friends, is my story.

My first clinical rotation was the lovely and ever popular internal medicine (in other words Gomerville in the inner-city Philadelphia hospital my roommate and I were assigned to). It was still our first week of the rotation when the senior resident grabbed my roommate and me and said we had someone to admit in the Emergency Room. So my roommate looked at me, and I looked at him and we headed off to our destination. Now was the ER on the first floor? Or was it the next level down on the back side of the building? Crap, I'll never find my way around this maze! I just told my roommate to keep the resident in sight because if we lost him we were screwed.

As we were trying to follow the wake of the senior resident gliding effortlessly through the halls with that magnificent long white coat flowing behind him (looking like Nicolas Cage in the that scene from *Face Off*), I proceeded to drop my patient list, EKG calipers, stethoscope, and Washington Manual (twice) out of my overstuffed short white jacket. Then we arrive. This is no Valhalla. The place is huge yet looks tiny with the incredible amount of people and stretchers crammed into any nook and cranny available. The resident stops at this stretcher that is unceremoniously parked in front of the main control desk. People are flying by every which way. It is total chaos. The senior resident tosses the chart at us. After quick review, the little lump under the sheet (head and all) turns out to be a 91-year-old man from a local nursing home.

I honestly don't even remember the chief complaint of the nursing home staff; but frankly it isn't really important to this story anyway. The patient is a demented, nonverbal, multi-system-involved train wreck. As *House of God* would put it – a typical gomer. After the resident does his physical exam, with the wide-eyed third-year students behind him nerdishly taking notes on the far superior resident's exam, he turns to me and says those fateful four words,

"Put on some gloves."

The words struck fear in my inner core. I looked over at my roommate with that "deer in the headlights" panic in my eyes. All I get back from him is the "thank God it isn't me" look. I froze. Again the resident says, "Put on some gloves" and pointed to the nearby cart where the typical assorted boxes were stacked. The sweat started to bead on my forehead and upper lip as I tried to squeeze into these incredibly tight blue gloves. I later found out they were a pair of small gloves. How was I to know they came in different sizes? I thought one size stretched to fit all.

So there I was. I was going to touch a patient. OK, remember the heart sounds, the location of each organ and how to percuss them. Don't forget the deep tendon reflexes, etc. Don't forget anything because you just know some pimping is coming. But as if it all happened in slow motion, the resident flips me this little blue and white packet, the size of a ketchup or mustard packet. With the same motion, he then whips back the sheet to expose this saggy, deflated 91- year-old ass. I catch the packet and look down. It reads "Surgilube." The instant knot in my stomach felt as though someone had just punched me in the pancreas.

He wanted me to do the rectal! Me!?!?!

But . . . but, I . . . I've never . . . Oh shit! Again my roommate gives me the "thank God it isn't me" look. *Bastard.* The resident grabs my white jacket and pulls me to the stretcher again dislodging my Washington Manual and patient list. My roommate quickly picks them up off the floor. *Gee, thanks. What a pal.* At this point my resident tries to calm me . . .

"Don't worry, he won't even know you're in there. Just lube up and stick 'em in."

Where the nerve came from I will never know, but I opened the Surgilube ketchup packet and totally lubed my right hand. Yes, I said right hand. As I said before, how was I supposed to know? With my left hand I grabbed his top sagging cheek and lifted to expose the Holy Grail. A quick look around the Emergency Room revealed that the chaos was still in high gear. The noise was deafening. I don't think anyone even knew we were there, even though we were right out in the open in front of everyone. There was medical staff, patients, family members, and on and on. I mean everyone.

So I pointed my fingers, took a deep breath and plunged those fingers right in. Immediately this demented, nonverbal, noncommunicative 91-year-old screams out at the top of his lungs . . .

"HEEEYYY, GIT YOUR FINGERS OUT OF MY ASS!!!!"

Yes, I froze again, with my fingers still firmly implanted in his ass. Just to remind me that my fingers were still indeed firmly implanted in his ass, the nonverbal 91-year-old gentlemen kindly repeated himself. Only this time louder . . .

"GIT YOUR FINGERS OUT OF MY ASS!!!!"

This time the cursory glance around the Emergency Room revealed not a single person moving. I don't recall any more noises and everyone now had their eyes squarely on this third-year medical student with his bulging short white coat, sweat pouring off his face, his totally lubed right hand with one finger in the elderly man's rectum doing his first rectal.

That's why I'll **NEVER** forget the Summer of '92. ✚

15

✚ A Medical Student Translation Guide for Patient Complaints

Yes, I'll try to lose weight!
=
I hope Burger King has the lunch menu up when I leave here.

Doctor, I have a very high tolerance of pain.
=
I am an absolute wimp who needs general anesthesia for a hangnail.

Yes, I exercise around the house.
=
I do nothing and the only sweat I get is with each bowel movement.

I only drink three or four beers a day.
=
I actually drink eight or nine beers a day; maybe 12 or 13.

I left my last doctor because he never listened to me.
=
No one ever listens to me; not even my friends or family, no one!
Doctor, are you listening?

By the way, Doc, what do think of that Viagra stuff?
=
My penis has been dead on arrival for years and I miss it so.

My cough is not due to my smoking!
=
Just give me the damn antibiotic so I can go get a smoke right outside the office!

I am not a drug seeker!
=
I am a drug seeker!

It hurts really bad in my back and neck and ankle and . . .
=
How about getting me on disability?

**I want the best medicine you've got,
my insurance pays for it.**
=
I want the best medicine you've got because I've got Medicaid.

Doctor, I only eat healthy foods!
=
I hope Burger King has the lunch menu up when I leave here.

The following occurred in my junior year on the OB service at a prominent hospital in Dallas in the 1960-61 academic year.

SYNCHRONIZED SWIMMING

"Joe Bob," a medical student famous for gaffes and wit, was charged with monitoring the labor of a teenage primigravida. His sole task was to call the resident when the patient was fully dilated.

As labor progressed, he snoozed until awakened by the patient's urgent request to visit the commode for a bowel movement. He obligingly helped her to a seat, whereupon she delivered a healthy, Apgar 9 male – *right into the toilet bowl.*

After hysterics and hysterical laughter subsided, the case was presented to the chairman of the department at OB Complications rounds the next week. The chairman was a notoriously ill-tempered taskmaster who demanded perfection from his charges and was fuming about the incident. The room was packed. Poor Joe Bob recited the awful facts as the chairman grew increasingly impatient with the unfolding scene. Finally the ordeal ended with Joe Bob slumped against the wall, overpowered by the steely gaze of the chairman, who boomed,

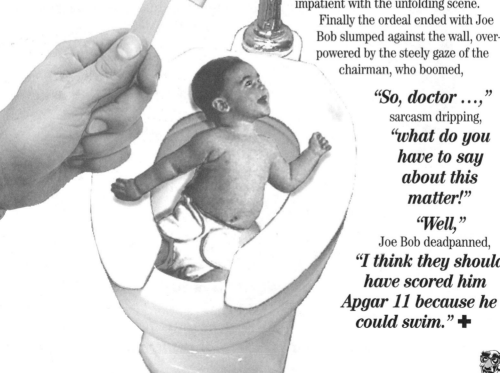

"So, doctor ...," sarcasm dripping, *"what do you have to say about this matter!"*

"Well," Joe Bob deadpanned, *"I think they should have scored him Apgar 11 because he could swim."* ✚

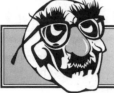

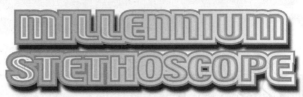

There I was, a third-year med student at the University of Kentucky, doing my first ER rotation. Recently, I had gotten to do chest compressions during a code and felt puffed up with pride when the nurse declared, *"I can feel a good femoral pulse."* On the other end of the spectrum, I had also seen the mother who brought her kid into the ER at 11 p.m. for his school immunizations because she had forgotten them and the child couldn't start school the next day without them (she was politely turned away and told to contact her child's pediatrician).

The good stuff, however, was yet to come. This shift, at about 2 a.m., we got notified of an **alpha trauma calldown**. All we knew was that it was a single-vehicle rollover accident with injuries.

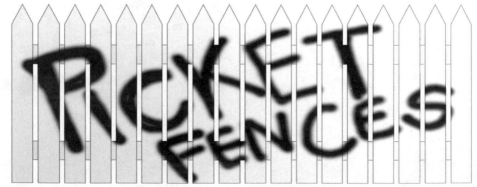

The trauma team gathered, we all "suited up" and soon the patient was wheeled into the trauma bay. He was a young male, 25 to 30 years old, conscious, and not really in very much distress. By his own admission, he had been getting high on pot all night with his buddies (*he didn't drink, he said, because he thought it would violate his probation*). After the party had wound down, he hopped into his pickup, drove faster than he ought to have, lost it in a turn, and was ejected from the vehicle as it rolled over.

Now imagine your arm in front of you, as though it were held in a sling. This man had a mossy, splintered 1 x 6 foot timber that went through the lower side of his forearm, exited through the top, continued on, went through his upper arm, and again exited the other side. There were rusty nails and grass all over this thing, but surprisingly little blood considering the amount of loose meat flapping around. He could even twitch his fingers a little.

It was time to act. After going through the ABCs of an emergency medical exam and looking in amazement at the wound itself, we proceeded with the secondary survey. We checked his other extremities.

"Does this hurt?," we asked.
"No," he responded.
We checked his cervical spine, *"Does this hurt?"* "No." *"Does THIS hurt?"* "No."
We checked his abdomen, we checked his pelvis. We log-rolled him to assess his back, and asked as we were palpating, *"Does this hurt?"* to which he replied, ***"I'm telling y'all, ain't nothing hurtin' on me 'cept my arm!"***

Incredibly enough, this guy had no broken bones, no major vascular injuries and there was very little neurological damage. Our friend, let's call him Bubba, barely avoided complying with the axiom: What's the last thing a dumb redneck says? ***"Hey y'all, watch this!"*** ✚

EDITOR'S NOTE: Do not try this at home. Bubba was lucky he didn't have the fence post jammed up his . . .

BOT FLY ON THE BRAIN

I picked the patient's chart up off the door. It read, **"Infected bug bite."** *"Alright! One I can handle,"* I thought. You see this was the first week of my first rotation of my third year of medical school and I was GREEN. I walked in still looking at the chart as I noticed that this "bug bite" had failed a first course of antibiotics . . . *Hmmm.*

The patient was your young surfer-dude type. He told me he had been traveling in Costa Rica two months before when he received this bite on his leg. Though he didn't see what bit him, he thought it was a mosquito because it itched like hell, and of course he had been scratching it.

The bite had been growing in size ever since and occasionally caused him a sharp pain, *like something was biting him.* He had seen my attending's partner two weeks prior and had received a course of antibiotics to cover for infection. There had been no improvement in the bite according to the surfer-dude. In fact, it had grown significantly. The bite mark itself was a small hole

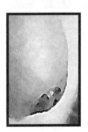

and there was a golf-ball sized raised mass underneath it. The mass had been growing up away from the bite – against gravity . . . *Hmmm.*

I asked him if he had squeezed it and if he had gotten anything out. This is when he broke down and confided in me his worst fears. *"Dude, I was so pissed at this bite. It hurts! I squeezed on it really hard one day and I got out what looked like a piece of segmented body or something. I think there's something growing in there! I can feel it moving sometimes!* **You got to get it out!"**

"Okay, relax, we won't send you home with just another course of antibiotics. Let me get my attending and we'll check it out." When I showed her the bite she responded, *"We're going in."*

A few minutes later with some local anesthesia and a scalpel my attending was cutting through the superficial layers of skin, then the fascia, then we saw it . . . a thick segmented body. I forgot myself and said out loud, *"Oh, man!"*

Our patient's head popped up instantly, *"What?!"* he asked. I looked over at him, realizing that all chances of me appearing professional to him had been shot and said, *"Did you declare this thing at customs?"*

"No way!" he responded, *"I knew there was something in there."*

My attending grabbed a pair of forceps and proceeded to remove a grub-like entity, 2 cm in length, 1 cm in diameter, tapered at either end, from the surfer-dude's leg. She didn't know what it was but she sent it off to pathology. I went home and asked a friend of mine who works in a travel clinic what the hell it was and she said, *"Bot Fly! Apparently they're pretty common. I'm so jealous you saw one! I've heard once you see one you see them all the time."*

I relayed this info to my attending and sure enough the pathology report came back, "Bot Fly." This story got around the office and my attending's partners were all a little jealous, too, that they had missed the Bot Fly Incident. It had certainly made my week.

On week two of my rotation I picked up a patient's chart off the door and it read, "Painful lump on back." *Hmmm . . .* I evaluated the patient, who had a lump growing for six weeks. It was becoming painful when he put pressure on it. I asked him if he had been traveling recently and he said, *"Why, yes, I got back from Costa Rica about two months ago. Do you think that has anything to do with it?"*

"Could you have been bitten on your back?" I asked.

"Well, yes, I was walking around without my shirt on!" Hmmm . . .

On examination, he had a golf-ball-size mass under a small hole! ***BINGO!*** The words of my friend came floating back to me, *"Once you see one you see them all the time."* Excitedly, I ran out to get my attending. I told her I had another Bot Fly for her. She, two of her partners, and a nurse that had missed the first Bot Fly, all returned to the patient's room with me. My patient was a little surprised at the entourage. I was a little mortified when they lifted up his shirt and immediately surmised "**Boil,**" turned and left. ✚

EDITOR'S NOTE: Only when you think you know a lot about medicine does something happen that makes you realize how little that amount actually is. **There Bot for the grace of God go I.**

RESPECT

I was a third-year medical student and he was a third-year OB-GYN resident when we crossed paths at the large county hospital in Texas. No, this is not a love story. There will not be an ending where we gazed into each other's eyes after a long night on call and fell into each other's arms in some sort of homo-erotic fantasy. No, this is a story of how some-one with low self-esteem immersed himself in the medical field, probably to gain power and pump up his ego and subsequently came very close to getting beaten to death – by me.

The obstetric rotation at this hospital had its good and bad points. The bad part was that the teaching wasn't the best because there was too much work to do. The good part, for medical students, was that even though they were going to kick your ass, you still would get a lot of deliveries. I chose this rotation because I liked the hands-on work. This place was nuts. I remember one time a resident delivering twins right in the triage room and one of them was breech. This was not malpractice because it was survival. Many of these patients were immigrants who would come into the country at the end of their pregnancy with no prenatal care and deliver their children on United States soil. It was a way, we assumed, that they could stay in the country. For a student, it was paradise. You could see anything and everything as long as you mentally survived the torture of the rotation.

The torture consisted of 5 a.m. rounds followed by watching surgical procedures or doing deliveries as they came. The work was endless and intermin-gled with it were lectures and pimping. The call, even for med students, was horrific and it was common to stay up all night and go 36 hours in a row. When you found a moment to rest, you either studied or slept. You never got enough of either.

The attendings were good old boys and rough. This is not to say that there weren't any female attendings. In fact, there were – they were rougher. They all had the same cowboy mentality as the men and usually beat up on students even harder.

That wasn't as bad as it sounds because you only interacted with attendings an hour or so a day. The bad part was that they really **22** brutalized the residents. Since sh%t rolls

downhill, each resident subsequently beat up on the person one rung below him or her. This is where I come in.

The rotation was going well for me until the last two weeks. Now I may not be an easy guy to boss around because, I admit, I don't take orders that well. I knew, however, that to survive I needed to put my head down and suck it up. Joe, the third-year resident, was a pretty boy. That is the best way to explain him, plain and simple. He was 6'2" tall, good looking, and married. Rumors about his affairs with other women were rampant. At first I didn't mind him or his attitude. I even tried to befriend him one late night on-call. Nothing worked because, for some reason, Joe just didn't like me.

Any night on-call with me, Joe would make me do unbelievable amounts of what we like to call **"scut" work**. This may be cleaning gross things up, doing blood draws on anyone and everyone, doing extra rounds, etc. It was obvious that he was sin-gling me out, but I put up with it. It got worse. Mature people wouldn't do this and if I was smart, I would have talked to him about his motives. The problem was that this attempt also could make things worse and kill my grade. So, I put up with it.

On one of my last nights on-call for the rota-tion, I was again paired up with my buddy Joe. He decided on his own to lay it on thick. He was full of himself and loved the power. Like the military, he had the hierarchy that was unbreakable. He beat me up with scut work and I couldn't do anything about it. I remember trying to catch a few minutes of sleep in the call room and each time he would overhead page me or beep me 10 minutes after I got into the room. He did that all night. The next day he laughed and laughed. There was nothing I could do as he just stared me down as I walked by to go home. He was the "man" – in his own mind.

At the end of the rotation I spoke with the head attending and chief of obstetrics at the hospital. I wanted to feel him out about my predicament without giving any names. He told me that if it was him, in this *hypothetical* situation, he would speak to the resident man-to-man, and lay it on the line. I knew what he was inferring. **I told you these guys were cowboys.**

The end finally came and luckily enough, I made it through the rotation and even got a decent grade. I was done with Joe. Unfortunately, my next rotation was in surgery at that same coun-ty hospital. This was an even better learning expe-rience than the OB-GYN rotation but I knew I would have to run into the egomaniac again. It was early in the surgery rotation when we were round-ing as a large group and walked by the obstetric floor. Out from the doors from the delivery area came Joe. He immediately saw me and stopped and started to stare. Pretty soon, like a 9-year-old kid, he started taunting me. *"Hey, buddy, how are you doing? They're not working you too hard are they? Are you tired?"*

I ignored him and looked away. He started in again, *"Come on, don't ignore me. Is my little friend tired? Why don't you do another OB rotation with me?"*

Finally the surgical group walked away. He was a dead man. I could tolerate his bullshit on the OB service because I had to, but now that I was off his rotation I felt I had no reason to take his crap. **I needed a plan.**

Okay, it wasn't a great plan. I decided I needed to tell him a few things in private. Though he was a big guy I wasn't afraid of him at all. I am only 5'7" tall but I was a collegiate wrestler and an all-American collegiate boxer. The funny thing is that Joe had known my history but I guess he didn't think it would come into play on his rotation. He was right – sort of.

By luck, a few days later I found Joe on the OB floor in a secluded hallway. All right, I admit it; I stalked him until I found him in the right place. As I walked toward him he chimed right in with the mocking. *"Hey, what are you doing here? Didn't you have enough last time?"*

"I just wanted to tell you a couple of things," I said. He actually stopped and listened inquisitively. *"When I was on your rotation you could haze me all you wanted. Now that I am on surgery you need to stop."*

His pompous facial expression showed that he didn't care. I continued, *"Because if you don't stop, I'm going to beat the living sh%t out of you!"* His expression turned to fear. *"And I'm not talking about a little beating either. I'm going to find you and beat you so bad that you won't be recognizable to anyone you know. You'd better have someone to help you, because once I start I'm not going to stop – until you're dead – you motherf*cker!"*

I thought the last part was a nice touch.

Joe's face turned to horror. Like a little boy, he almost started to cry and said *"Why, what did I do?"*

I guess he wasn't so tough after all. *"You know what you did. Don't talk to me or look at me again because you are going to pay with your life!"*

With that statement another OB resident walked through the double-doors, which tipped me off that it was time to leave. As I went past him through those same doors, I heard Joe almost crying *"I can't believe this! I can't believe this!"* As I walked down and got to the end of the hallway, I heard the other resident pop his head out of the double-doors and scream (*and this is no lie*),

"HEY! HEY! SHOW SOME RESPECT!"

Respect? I just continued to walk and laugh to myself. ***Respect is earned. Crying in the hallway after torturing poor medical students doesn't get respect. You need to respect others in order for them to respect you.*** **Both of those residents were losers.** They are the stereotypical cocky doctors that give all of us a bad name. I am sure they never changed.

The next day in the Dean of Medicine's office (*You didn't think I got away with it?*), I thought to myself, *Maybe this wasn't the best plan.* I apologized to the dean and said what I had to so as not to get into too much trouble. I was made to see another bigwig in OB who demanded I get counseling for anger control.

I agreed, at the moment, to everything and have never gotten any permanent blotches on my record. I shortened this part of the story because it isn't as fun as the rest. The truth is that they wanted me to screw up again so they could run my ass out of the school. I never did. What I did do was this. Every time I saw Joe, whether in the parking lot or the hall, I would just stand there and stare at him. Turning the tables on him was worth it all. *For all he knew, I was psychotic.* Suffice it to say, he never said a word to me again. In fact, he would just put his head down and walk away. I should have, but never did, scream,

HEY! HEY! SHOW SOME RESPECT! ✚

23

Perc or Drip?

During my emergency department rotations as a PA (physician assistant) student, I was working with my preceptor in a small, rural town.

A short 30-year-old female and her significant other walked into the center of this little ER and she announced *"I have chest pain!"* This is big news in a small hospital and everybody around began to get their game faces on. After I looked at the patient, I turned to one of the nurses next to me and in my inner-city sarcastic "expertise" said *"Not!"* I was a little jaded since I had been an RN in a Level I trauma center for a long time and acquired what you would call a sixth sense of suspicion.

The patient proceeded to tell us that they were traveling through Arizona from California and she had taken two "nitros" about four hours apart without any relief of the pain. She had a past medical history of a neurological problem as her only significant marker. Her EKG, however, did look markedly abnormal but without the tombstone ST elevations that would make us start grabbing the thrombolytics.

My preceptor happened by at this time while I was muttering doubt about this patient's history. She also noticed my skepticism. She was a wonderful teacher and very compassionate. Obviously this is a quality I needed to acquire. *Unlearning some of my old baggage is not that easy.* She subsequently helped me work up the patient and soon I began to feel very ashamed of my "attitude."

The funny thing is that even though we gave the patient an appropriate amount of morphine to quell her cardiac pain, our lady kept requesting some Percodan.

The couple kept mumbling the whole time how "stupid" we were when she wasn't getting her "drug of choice." *I guess they thought it was a restaurant where they could order off the menu.* When we finished the workup, my preceptor determined that she had to be admitted to rule out a potential myocardial infarction. In order to get a better grasp of her

THOSE DARN NARC SEEKERS

"neurologic disorder," attempts were made to reach her physician in California.

During this time the patient kept insisting that she needed the Percodan for her pain. *"I NEED MY MEDS!"* she would scream. We had a heck of a time getting that complaint under control. On a personal level, I kept admonishing myself that I was no longer an inner-city nurse but a PA now and therefore had to view patient's complaints in a more professional manner.

I finished up the entire history and physical exam and then went off to a separate room to dictate it.

When I returned to the ER, my preceptor as well as the entire ER staff began laughing and bowing to me. It seems that while I was off dictating, the patient had become more agitated and grew angry while demanding more Percodan. Not getting the drug fast enough for her liking, she totally lost control. With one swift move, she finally tore out her IV and walked out of the hospital dripping blood. You could follow her trail like bread crumbs and probably find her and her husband at the next hospital a few towns away.

The truth finally came out when her neurologist in California called back and promptly filled us in on how this patient travels to small towns using her abnormal EKG as her calling card. Since she had had heart surgery as a child her EKG was always abnormal. She would throw in a neurological disorder hoping to make her case sound more serious and subsequently convince small town doctors to snow her with narcotics.

There are some things that my past experience has shown me. First, never get too excited even if it is chest pain and second, always trust your sixth sense. In a complete about-face, my preceptor told me I taught her a lesson and that she would never doubt my call about drug-seeking patients again.

What can I say, it's a gift. ✚

MY FAVORITE MUNCHAUSEN

Munchausen Syndrome was named after Baron Von Munchausen who always lied and told tall tales (John Neville, Uma Thurman, and Eric Idle starred in The Adventures of Baron Munchausen). *The Baron has many stories, he even has his own websites.*

NOTE: *The editors find the* **Munchausen Syndrome** *intriguing in an odd way. Publishing these stories may aid some physicians to diagnose these patients with a factitious disorder. We in no way want to make fun of people with psychiatric disorders. Munchausen By Proxy is child abuse and we will not use or publish any of those stories for that reason.*

This **MY FAVORITE MUNCHAUSEN** *comes from the February 2001 edition of the* Annals of Plastic Surgery.

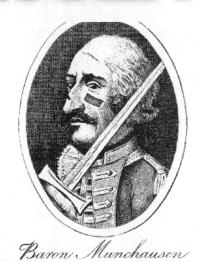

Baron Munchausen

A 26-year-old whom we will call "Lymphedema Lucy," to give her a personality, kept coming into hospitals for repeat edisodes of septicemia for a huge ulceration on her left lower leg. After being seen by at least five or six different hospitals during the past five years, it was apparent that no one could find the cause of Lucy's problem. No matter what treatment was given, her ulcerations would never heal. Her leg became massive in size and she could no longer ambulate.

Multiple invasive diagnostic procedures were performed, but Lucy could find no help. Interestingly enough, the lymphedema always kept starting around 10 cm from the groin region. Lucy was getting frustrated and began requesting amputation of the entire limb to solve all her problems. Astute physicians had factitious disorder in their differential all along. With a team of psychiatrists now involved, Lucy fessed up. It is amazing what secretly placing a plastic cord around your leg for five years can do to your skin.

We will never know exactly why "Lymphedema Lucy" felt so inclined to put a tourniquet around her thigh and make her leg look like an old duffel bag. The authors felt maybe the pressure of adulthood and the need to lead an independent life may have been the cause. Or maybe the care of her ailing father years earlier and then his eventually death played a part? Nonetheless, Lucy received major reconstruction of her leg, which only added to the incredible financial strain that she had placed on the medical system for her care. ✚

De Fontaine S, Van Geertruyden, Preudíhomme X, et al. "Munchausen Syndrome." Ann Plast Surg *2001;46:153-58.*

MOODY

So there I was, a third-year medical student on my psychiatry rotation. Psychiatry seemed to come easy to me, and I found myself actually enjoying it. I was assigned once a week to a doctor that worked with geriatric psychiatric issues. He was a very pleasant individual, but a little difficult to understand at times. He was of Asian descent (I am not really sure where exactly) and he had a rather thick accent. He worked closely with one of the local nursing homes and had to do rounds one week. I worked with him.

So there we were, the patient was not eating and having homicidal ideations. The doctor asked the nurse to bring her into the lunchroom, as she had a roommate. The doctor, the third-year resident, the nursing home resident, and I sat at a small table on the side of the room farthest from the door. The room echoed terribly, and to make matters worse, there was the noise of the air conditioning and the ice machine.

"Sally" was in her late eighties, pleasant, in a wheelchair, and of course, very hard of hearing.

We asked her a few questions, and after repeating multiple times, tried writing. We got some mumbled answers, and eventually got her to talk without us having to write our questions. We went on asking her questions about what was wrong, etc.

"How's your mood?" asked the doctor, in his thick accent.

"HUH?" she replied.

"How's your mood?" he replied, leaning in closer to her.

There was a pause, and Sally got this very puzzled look on her face. The doctor starts talking to the resident when Sally blurts out, *"I don't eat wood."* At that point, I couldn't help it and I let out a muffled laugh. The resident and doctor both must not have heard her because I got the weirdest look from both of them. I quickly explained what had happened, and both the resident and doctor laughed before continuing with the interview. I just couldn't help but try to put myself in Sally's position. Here are three strangers, and one is asking her if she eats wood. ✦

TRUE TALES OF MISTAKEN IDENTITY

Patients in teaching hospitals are seen and evaluated by so many doctors and other health professionals on a daily basis that it's understandable that they get some of us mixed up. As a medical student, I've come to accept this. The most frequent misnomer applied to me (typically by an older, male patient) is **"nurse"** (*which wouldn't bother me at all if I'd ever heard of a male student being addressed this way*). Some of my patients, however, have gotten even more creative.

One patient that I took care of on an internal medicine service decided that I was her **"special angel"** – in part because of my blond hair and in part, I'm guessing, because the resident had grown bored with her days before her discharge, rendering me her primary caregiver. While I was doing my psychiatry rotation, another patient announced that I looked like a **"magical elf,"** and wanted to know where my wand was. At that point I guess I should have taken out my penlight and waved it over his head. Maybe I could have "cured" him.

By far the most amusing case of mistaken identity occurred during my day seeing patients at the county jail. This was located on the top few floors of a tall municipal building outside Boston. The

infirmary was a bleak, institutional room with one space walled off for seeing patients. Toward the end of the morning, I was wandering around the room trying not to touch anything (*the electrostatic shocks from the plastic and metal furniture were almost enough to defibrillate me*), waiting for the doctor to emerge from the exam area. Across the room from me, the next patient was waiting. He was a big, heavyset African-American man in his prison-issued jumpsuit. At one point I saw him motion the nurse toward him, but I couldn't hear their conversation. Later, the nurse filled me in:

Inmate: *"Who is that girl over there?"* (motions toward me)

Nurse: *"She's a medical student. She's with Dr. Smith today."*

Inmate: *"She scares me. (pause) Is she an albino or something?"*

Nurse: *"No, I think she just has blond hair. (pause) She doesn't have to come in if you don't want her to."*

Inmate: (Shakes head vigorously)

Needless to say, I didn't get to examine that patient. However, if I ever meet him in a dark alley, I guess we know which one of us will start running first. ✦

ANOMALY

It was the end of my sixth month of medical school and it was getting old already. The same routine of going to classes, lab sessions, or working with the microscope was monotonous. I wanted to be a real doctor and not a professional student. Each night was spent studying for three to five hours. Each morning the same faces were sitting in the same seats in the same lecture hall. Some were ass kissers. Some were bullshitters. The only reprieve, I thought, was the anatomy lab.

At first, the anatomy class was exciting. A group of four would receive their "body" at the start of the year and dissect it over the next six months. Ours had tattoos on his forearm so he was affectionately named Popeye. By the end we were down to bare bones and tendons. Initially, the class gave us a chance to joke around. It sounds worse than it was, but it was a way for medical students to blow off steam. Sure it was gallows humor but it was fun. We did respect the dead but we also joked around. That was in the beginning. After a few months, however, we just wanted to be done with it. The tests were hands-on practicals as well as the basic memorization written tests. We prepared for this, not only by the normal dissection practices, but also by going to small lectures. These were held in tucked-away classrooms containing around thirty first-year medical students. Twice a week we had to present our findings in the lab to the rest of the class. An anatomist professor would preside over it but the student would do most of the work presenting.

These side sessions soon became extremely tedious as well. Although they were needed and classroom attendance was mandatory, they soon became draining as well. I remember, like it was yesterday, the time I was to present on the renal system. The kidney was my topic and I had to stand up and draw pictures and discuss all the functions of this most mundane system. The problem on this day, however, was that I was too mentally exhausted to prepare. An hour before the side session I was eating a salad in lunch when it hit me. My classmates were in a solemn mood as we talked about life, medicine, and school in general. I knew that after this break we all would walk to the classroom to watch me do my show. I, however, had no show to give . . . until I looked in my salad dish. There lay a perfect kidney bean with a remnant of its skin hanging down.

Hell, it looked a miniature kidney (with a ureter attached)!

After sneaking it into a napkin, I stuck it into my pocket and walked with the rest of my classmates. No one saw what I did. After we arrived, the teacher gave his introduction to the subject and called me up to present. I began stating that instead of doing the usual routine, I was going to spend my time discussing an amazing discovery. I brought the napkin and raised the small kidney bean.

"You have before you an anomaly. Our cadaver seemed to have an abnormal kidney. One side was normal and the other had shrunk due to either disease, non-use, or a congenital problem. I know it is wrong to take the organ out of the lab, but you all need to see the miniature kidney and its very small ureter."

For the first time in a while, the students seemed awake after their luncheon slumber. Their eyes were like saucers as I walked around and showed each and every one of them the pale and decayed organ (or salad condiment). No one caught on, not even the teacher.

I walked up to the head of the classroom again and made up some more crap about why it could be so small. Then, after a few seconds' delay and an uncomfortable silence, I tossed the kidney bean up in the air around four feet and caught it in my mouth and ate it. *"Oh my God!"* one student said. No one else said a word as the uncomfortable silence continued. The teacher didn't even say anything but instead maintained a very strained and constipated look on his face. At that point I said *"thank you"* and walked back to my seat.

The grumblings began to start as I hit my chair and the teacher got up to walk toward me. It was only then that my classmates, who had been sitting next to me at lunch, realized what the truth was and started laughing their asses off. Knowing that I was soon to get into major trouble, I confessed my sins to everyone. The teacher was not pleased and many of the other students were also pissed off. I was not suspended, but for the rest of the semester I was treated with a little disdain and a lot of disgust by many of my peers. I now had a reputation. An anomaly is a rare abnormality out of the norm. I, like my miniature kidney, was now the anomaly of medical school. ✚

FUBIGMI %#*@¢!

We called him the Cone, or Cal Conehead because it was the early eighties and he related to the house staff like an extraterrestrial. He was the chief of the Department of Medicine at a large midwestern academic hospital and he occasionally would come down from his ivory tower to enlighten our early morning intake rounds on the wards. His wisdom was worthless to us, and after decades without any patient contact, he could no longer connect with our lives. But he was a likeable fellow, and so we referred to him not derogatorily but in a cynically affectionate way as *"The Cone."* I was a fourth-year medical student like eight or ten others. We were assembled in a circle outside a patient's room with our medical resident and two medical interns one predawn morning late in the academic year when *The Cone* arrived unexpectedly. It had been a brutal night on-call for many of us who were still clad in wrinkled scrubs and in need of a shower and a shave (even the women), not to mention rest. To make matters worse, we had recently learned where we had matched to do our internships the upcoming July, and we all had fulminant cases of **FUBIGMI** (F%ck You, Buddy. I Got My Internship). This made it safe to behave a little less submissively than usual.

The Cone began lecturing profusely and irrelevantly about the difference between "people doctors" and "thing doctors." Being Chief of Medicine, *The Cone* had a prejudice against surgical types who he called "thing doctors," a derogatory term for a physician who viewed his patients as a bag of removable things (organs). Internists, by contrast, we were told, were "people doctors" because of their more integrated and holistic view of the patient as an entity comprised of interrelated physical and mental systems.

We were each forced to answer in turn if we were on our way to becoming "people doctors" or "thing doctors," an exercise in humiliation for the surgeons-to-be amongst us. Begrudgingly, we answered in turn, forced to call ourselves "thing doctors" or "people doctors." The best answer came from the fourth-year medical student on his way to becoming a neurosurgeon with the worst case of **FUBIGMI** ever witnessed at our institution. When his turn came, he proudly announced, *"Dr. Cone, I'm not gonna be a people doctor or a thing doctor. I'm gonna be a doctor who turns people into things!"* We laughed so hard, one guy wet himself and another dropped his clipboard. *The Cone* reportedly stopped rounding with post-match students thereafter. ✚

EDITOR'S NOTE: *Let's hope this neurosurgeon doesn't get patients that PITH him off or they will be wearing drool buckets.*

MAKE YOUR QUESTIONS CLEAR

As a fourth-year medical student on my gynecological rotation I was faced with a twenty-ish patient whose chief complaint was, "My funk do smell." Examination of the patient and her vaginal discharge made it obvious that I was dealing with a sexually transmitted disease.

I asked, *"Are you sexually active?"* to which she replied, rather indignantly, *"NO!!"*

I repeated my question, feeling perhaps that she had misunderstood, yet the answer was still, *"NO!!"*

Confused, I then gently asked, *"When was the last time that you had sex?"*

Her answer then was straightforwardly delivered as, *"Last Friday."*

"I thought you just told me that you are not sexually active?" I exclaimed, to which she answered, *"I'm not, I just lay there."* ✚

EDITOR'S NOTE: *I had always thought this was a joke or an urban legend. Our reader signed off that this was "absolutely true" and happened to him.*

28

Escapee

I was a wet-behind-the-ears third-year medical student on my trauma surgery rotation. One afternoon, I was relishing the opportunity to put in a central line on a comatose ICU patient. When I had finished, it was close to our usual check-out time, so I looked around expecting to see the other trauma team members. Not only were they all missing, but so were several ICU nurses. I could not imagine what sort of emergency would require the attention of the entire trauma team and nurses without setting off my pager as well.

As it turns out, one of our patients had gone AWOL.

The patient was a young man who had walked into the ED last night after being shot in the head. I repeat: he **WALKED** into the ED on his own, after being **SHOT IN THE HEAD**. He also had fractures of two cervical vertebrae. The young man had been in the ICU, with a neck brace on, when several police officers and FBI agents came looking for him. When he heard that they were there, he got out of bed, removed his neck brace and IVs, and ran, stark naked, out of the hospital. They finally caught him in the hospital parking lot, trying to find an unlocked car in which to make his getaway. Needless to say, he had a police guard posted on him continuously until he was discharged. ✚

EVERYONE NEEDS | A NICKNAME

I was a third-year medical student on my OB rotation. The usual crowd was assembled in the delivery room as my buddy Marc, a fellow MS3, was preparing to inject local anesthesia into the perineum of an immediately pre-delivery mother-to-be who was about to receive her episiotomy. Also present in the room were two more students, an intern, a resident, the chief resident, the expectant father, and three nurses.

With Mom in the lithotomy position, legs spread wide, Marc approached her with the syringe filled with lidocaine. He was visibly nervous, having never done this before, and being where he was between this woman's gaping legs and in the presence of so many people only added to his burden.

His tension was infectious, and the room was completely quiet for a moment as Marc brought the needle closer to its intended target.

The mood changed immediately when Marc perfunctorily announced to the patient and everyone else present that she was about to feel,

"a little prick."

Everyone, even the mother, was laughing at Marc, who had that day inadvertently coined his own new nickname. ✚

Going NUTS in Anatomy Lab

Our days as medical students in the anatomy lab had become terribly monotonous. Certain days were exciting . . . slicing through layers of fascia, digging around in the abdomen, and sawing through the skull. But most days were the same old thing . . . following an artery or nerve through its twists and turns or delicately scraping fat from thin muscle fibers. As the days went by, my good friend and I felt the need to spice things up. We found a metal nut that had become unscrewed from the metal cadaver tank and thought we'd do a little experiment. *Medicine is supposed to be evidence-based, right?*

We hadn't yet dissected the uterus, so using the handle of a scalpel, we carefully pushed the nut up into the uterus of our dear Rosemary. A few more boring weeks passed until we began studying the reproductive system. Finally, the day came when we were told to dissect the uterus. My friend and I watched in anticipation over the body as a classmate sawed down Rosemary's midline into the uterus. As the uterus split in half, we could see the student's jaw drop. Sitting smack dab in the middle of the posterior wall of the uterus was a nice shiny nut.

Our classmate screamed, *"I found a nut; I found a nut!"* Classmates began gathering around the dissection table to witness the "discovery." Within seconds, the entire class was gathered around. Of course, everyone initially thought Rosemary had a testicle, which would have been a pretty cool finding, but when they realized it was a metal "nut," the excitement in the room grew out of control. We had seen prosthetic knees, pacemakers, and even an "old-school" penis pump, but nothing compared to this discovery!

Before long, the sea of medical students parted as the teaching assistant approached the body. His face lit up; you could see the "I'm gonna get published with this discovery" sparkle in his eyes. With amazement he proclaimed, *"I've never seen anything like this. Don't touch it. Leave it in its natural state."*

As he ran out of the room, my friend and I began to worry. We knew where he was going; this whole adventure was beginning to get carried away. Lab work seemed boring, but flipping burgers at McDonald's after getting expelled from med school would be even worse. Suddenly the lab door flew open and the crowd was silenced. The God of Anatomy had just entered. The professor was in the lead with the teaching assistant kissing his rear end. As the professor approached the body, my friend and I were shaking in fear. *It was too late to say anything now!* We just held our breath in hopes that the whole ordeal would end quickly. Our future in medicine was quickly fading while the scent of McDonald's fries filled our minds. The professor examined the nut, scratched his chin, and stated, *"I have read several publications on this matter. This is definitely not the first finding of this sort. Whether it be a sexual fetish or a migration from another part of the body, there are scientific explanations for such a finding."*

Once the professor was gone, we let out a sigh of relief and explained to our classmates the true origin of "the nut." For some reason, the days following the "discovery" weren't so boring anymore! We were just thankful to be handling fatty human muscles rather than fatty hamburger patties! ✚

Cracking (Up) the Code

I am a fourth-year medical student currently (*and mercifully*) finishing up my last few rotations at a Big Academic Center Hospital in Boston. My colleagues and I were interrupted in the middle of SICU (Surgical Intensive Care Unit) rounds last week by one of the nurses, who wanted to tell us about the new code protocol.

She explained to us that next time one of us (*obviously not me*) responded to a code, we would be asked as we arrived whether or not we would be leading the code. If the answer was yes, we would be immediately be handed a ring-bound collection of laminated green cards upon which were printed the ACLS (Advanced Cardiac Life Support) algorithms. These cards, she explained as we passed them around, would serve two purposes: to identify the code leader, and to help him or her with the algorithms (*not that any of our residents would EVER forget such a thing*).

As soon as she left, we started thinking about what other means might be used to identify the code leader in the event that the green cards were misplaced. Here are some of the alternatives we envisioned:

1. A beanie cap with a propeller on top. Clearly the silliest of the options, this would also be the most unmistakable, visible even from the medical student's vantage point (*which tends to be somewhere out in the hall*).

2. A large red clown nose. This would not only identify the code leader, but also, if it squeaked loudly enough, aid him or her in attracting the attention of other code responders at critical points in the resuscitation (*such as when the defibrillator is about to discharge*).

3. A "Miss America"–style satin sash emblazoned with "Code Leader" in cursive lettering. Though it might be cumbersome to drape properly during the middle of a code, this is definitely the most photogenic of the options.

4. A crown and scepter. These would undoubtedly help instill the code leader with the confidence and authority necessary to perform his duties. In a pinch, the scepter could also be used to deliver precordial thumps.

5. A coach's whistle. Visually subtle, this little tool would be indispensable in calling attention to "code fouls," such as catheterizing the carotid artery, intubating the esophagus, or successfully resuscitating a patient who was DNR (*oops*). ✚

Medical Memories from the
UNIVERSITY STATE PEN

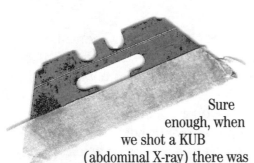

Our university hospital treated the prisoners from the State Pen. We had a prison unit complete with guards and sliding barred doors that we had to pass through in order to make rounds.

The prisoners really liked the unit; it had private rooms, three square meals a day, color TV, etc. They figured out a clever way to get admitted: they would place a piece of masking tape over the edge of a single-edge razor blade and then swallow the razor blade. Then they informed the guards, who brought them to the ER.

Sure enough, when we shot a KUB (abdominal X-ray) there was a razor blade in the stomach. We would then admit them for observation until they passed the razor blade. We eventually caught on.

One night I was in the ER, as a third-year student, and one of these guys came in. We had just figured out what the prisoners were doing, but they didn't know yet. The new protocol was to drop an NG (nasogastric) tube, and if there was no blood, send them back to the jailhouse.

Well, I dutifully snaked the tube down, and there was no blood that couldn't be accounted for by my root-hogging this tube through his nose. I told the guy he was being sent back to the big house.

Thank God for the prison guards, because this guy went totally ballistic. He lunged at me, but the guards caught him by the arms. Then he tried to reach out with his foot and kick me, but I managed to dance away. Unfortunately, I was not out of projectile range and he hit my tie with a nice, juicy loogie.

They subsequently decided to up the ante: they unwound their bed springs and stabbed themselves in the abdomen. One guy came in with this piece of wire in his belly that was twitching at his pulse rate. *I was sooooo tempted to tell him to come back when it was an inch deeper.*

✛

I was a third-year medical student doing my first clinical rotation – Psychiatry Consult Service. My classmate and I were sent to do a mental status exam on a patient. We were asking the standard questions to determine if our confused elderly man had concrete or abstract reasoning – *"What is the same about a dog and a horse?"* and *"a truck and a car?"*

We had been taught that depressed patients don't really care if they can't answer questions, but that those with organic brain syndromes will sometimes try to change the subject to distract the examiner and obfuscate our ability to detect their deficits.

So, this cheerful old man asked my classmate – *"Now, son, let me ask you one. Do you know the difference between silk curtains and toilet paper?"*

Thinking this was a setup for a joke,

the other student answered,

"No, what?"

The response – *"Well, don't come to my house!!!!"* He got full credit for that answer. ✚

Night Stick

When I was a fourth-year medical student on the surgical service, we admitted a 22-year-old woman for persistent rectal bleeding. Nothing that her primary care doctor tried helped. Her radiological studies were all negative. While inhouse, she continued to bleed daily. We actually suspected Munchausen Syndrome but needed a way to prove it. . . .

. . . We decided to mix a fluorescent dye in with her lidocaine jelly (which we were giving her for the anal discomfort). We then sneaked into her room in the middle of the night with a black light. This is what is used to make those old Elvis posters glow, etc.

To our disgust, her pencils lit up!!!

Needless to say, she was discharged in the morning. ✚

EDITOR'S NOTE – Now I know what the Number 2 means on the pencil!

It was the first week of my fourth year of medical school. I was assigned to do a one-week rotation on the Urology Service. *Piece of cake*, I thought to myself. No one expects you to know anything during a one-week rotation. Good thing, too, since despite three years of medical school, I still didn't know jack about the male genital/prostate exam. It's not my fault; it's a gender thing. Girl students can practice on girl patients, no problem. Girl students may not practice on boy patients, full stop. That is, of course, until you start your one-week Urology rotation, then miraculously you're supposed to know all about it. *Hey, no problem, I read the book . . .*

The first couple of days were easy: morning conferences and then stand around in surgery plastered against the wall out of the way. I wasn't asked to scrub in, I wasn't even pimped. Like I said, no one expects you to know anything on a one-week rotation. If you're lucky, they don't even learn your name.

Unfortunately, my comfortable anonymity ended Wednesday afternoon, Clinic Day. The patient was a 60-year-old man with prostate cancer successfully treated with radiation therapy the previous year. He was at the clinic for a routine every third month surveillance visit and all he needed was a PSA (blood test for prostate cancer) and a DRE (digital rectal exam).

Easy, I thought, *I can pull this one off.* I had been told ahead of time not to do the

THE K-Y THAT GOT AWAY

prostate exam until the resident was in the room. This way the patient only has to drop his drawers once. So, I gathered all the other information and presented him to the chief resident. *So far, so good.*

We entered the room and the chief handed me a glove and took one herself. She put K-Y jelly on her finger and handed me the rest of the packet. After informing the patient that he was getting *"two for one today,"* she performed the rectal exam and told me to do the same and tell her what I felt. On my turn I noted good tone, stool in vault and a small, firm but smooth prostate gland. No, there were no nodularities and yes it was symmetric. She nodded. *Yes!*, I thought. First impressions are so important.

Triumphantly, I withdrew my finger and pulled the glove off and as I did a spray of K-Y jelly flew across the room. I looked over at the chief and noted two large, brown-streaked globs of K-Y clinging to her cheek. Disturbingly, she did not raise her hand to remove the jelly. She just looked at me, brow furrowed, shaking her head in disbelief as if she was thinking, *"And why did God send you to me today?"*

Surprisingly, I did pass my Urology rotation. Or maybe not so surprisingly since the chief, I'm sure, didn't want me anywhere near her Urology Clinic ever again.

✦

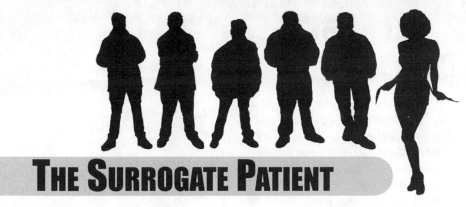

THE SURROGATE PATIENT

As a medical student in Philadelphia, the approach of my OB-GYN rotation filled me with nervous anticipation. At this early stage in our careers, facing the utter dread of being unmasked by a patient as the phony you knew you were, the idea of "clinical rotations" were anxiety-provoking anyway. Add to the mix the awkwardness of the female pelvic exam and our group had more nervous energy than Robin Williams on amphetamines.

In order to prepare us for the experience, my school enlisted the aid of "Surrogate Patients" for the third years to practice the art of the pelvic exam. The group of around thirty students met at the hospital clinic and were divided into groups of six, each with a preceptor and a "patient." **The patients (whom we learned were paid handsomely by the school for their services) were made up of five militant, angry-appearing, army-boot-wearing 200-lb. women with haircuts like Drew Carey. The sixth was a very attractive woman in her mid-twenties.** I had very mixed feelings when I was assigned to the latter. It was hard enough to try and be cool about this admittedly terrifying situation, but to have the woman be someone you could envision yourself hitting on at a bar?!?

Luck would have it that among my group of all male fellow classmates, I was chosen to go first. **The woman/patient apparently felt it would be helpful to "coach" me through the experience and let me know how things felt from her end.** She went through the basics, such as not to say the breasts *"FEEL FINE"* or *"GOOD,"* but *"Your EXAM is NORMAL and HEALTHY"* was acceptable. This I handled with remarkable aplomb. Then came the pelvic exam.

The speculum portion of the exam went well, as I went slowly and steadied my shaking hand. **It did not help matters that the room was about 90 degrees, and I could feel the perspiration dripping down my face.** The next part was the bimanual exam. She coached on, *"Now examine my ovaries, you should be able to palpate my ovaries, because I'm thin."* My fear of somehow being sexually aroused by the experience was dissipating and I was concentrating with all the intensity I could muster to seem like I knew what I was doing. *"There, do you feel my ovary?"* I was not sure. I kept on adjusting the positioning of my hands in order to perfect my technique during this unique opportunity. With growing confidence, I exclaim,
"Yes! I think I have it!"
This high point was brief as my patient/coach whispered *"That's good. Now please take your thumb off of my clitoris."* With the reaction time of someone who just grabbed a hot potato, I yanked my hands out of the patient and fell backwards out of my chair as if I had been shot out of a cannon, to the raucous laughter of my classmates and preceptor.

I've wondered since this experience what kind of woman volunteers to subject her privates for the awkward fumblings of a doctor in training. Maybe they feel that they are contributing to the medical community. But perhaps it is simply to put a cocksure medical student in his place.

✦

ZINGO!

Back in my medical school days I recall sitting and listening to seemingly endless lectures from faculty members in the huge tiered classroom that was my world for years one and two. We were like 212 large sponges absorbing every bit of knowledge, useful or useless, that was thrown our way. Sitting in plastic chairs in the dark room, lit only by the lecturer's slides (in the pre–Power Point era), we often struggled for ways to maintain interest and to basically stay awake.

We had our share of the "big ones," anatomy, physiology, biochemistry et al. But along with those, thrown in by well-intentioned curriculum engineers, were the once a week "blow offs" like public health and medical jurisprudence. Even the most energetic *(in other words, the ass kissers)* of the 212 would be hard-pressed to stay conscious during one of these snore fests! So we, the most innovative of the 212, came up with a way to hold interest while these PhD's droned on about matters that would bore the most hardcore member of the NIH.

Say hello to Lecture Hall Zingo! Zingo was a game that anyone who was so inclined could play. It was very much like its semi-namesake Bingo. We would draw up little cardboard playing cards and for a mere dollar *(remember, we were medical students)* one could purchase a card.

Instead of a grid of random numbers, we placed in each box the name of one of our classmates. Of course, these students had no idea they were actually game pieces in our little adventure. No, these were the most special of the 212! These were the few, the proud, the **PAINS IN THE ASS!** You know whom I mean. Every class has them. These were the guys and girls who just liked to hear the sound of their own voices and who would ask inane questions or make ridiculously obvious comments for no good reason at all. We had roughly 20 of these and I loved every one of them. *For without them, we would never have had Zingo!*

Anytime one of the Zingo-ites bleated out a question or comment, whoever had them on their card would scratch an X over their name. It may have taken a few lectures or maybe even a few days, but when a card holder had a vertical, horizontal, or diagonal line covered by X's he was a potential winner. I use the word "potential" here since simply having a winning card was only the first step in collecting the pot of Zingo money. To actually collect, the winner had to yell out the word ZINGO so that all in the room could hear it. This made for some of the funniest moments I will ever remember in class. Well, except for shooting orange seeds at the lecturer and scoring points for accuracy, but that will have to wait for another article. ✚

QUE?

I was a lowly third-year medical student doing one of those God-awful, Saturday morning rotations which were "beneficial" for my education and allowed me to "appreciate the patient-disease continuum." My torturous, lazy internal medicine intern was busy flirting with the ward clerk and I was hastily doing a history and physical on a middle-aged Hispanic man who spoke very little English. The history was endless and by now my time off had begun and I was still standing there in this dingy city hospital room. I began to rush through the review of systems.

"Have you had heart disease?"
"Que?"

I pointed to my heart.

"Problem here?" I asked helpfully.

"NO, no" he replied as he looked confusedly at my breasts.

"OK, anemia, convulsions, cancer, smoking?" I asked. "You have a cough. How about TB?"

"What? Why do you want to know that?"

I groaned. I would be here until Sunday. "Look you really ought to tell me. Do you know anyone with TB?"

He shrugged his shoulders. "Yes, I like to watch sometimes. Not too much, you know."

Needless to say, his review of systems was actually negative. ✚

I COULD SURE USE SOME FRESH AIR

Gosh darn dentists. Our Munchausen recently stated she had a procedure resulting in terrible complications. "Ariel" had her tooth extracted in another state and soon developed an abscess under her chin. She was 30 years old and worked as an emergency medical technician. For ten weeks, Ariel dealt with pain and swelling. Oral antibiotics didn't seem to help and she was subsequently hospitalized in order to administer IV antibiotics. Her neck was drained and a tracheostomy was performed. Nothing seemed to help. Things were getting worse when our heroes, who reported this tale in the journal of ENT, received Ariel under their care. Her cellulitis was so bad that air was actually getting under the skin.

Ariel was on three antibiotics and one antifungal medication when the authors received her care. The whole right side of her face was extremely swollen and the air had traveled under the skin from her right eye all the way to her jaw and neck. The pain was extraordinary.

When she was first admitted there was no fever. Her white count was normal. CT scan showed extensive air all throughout the head and neck. A bone scan showed uptake in the right maxilla (below the right eye). Yet, with all the money spent on finding a cause for this interesting presentation, the answer still eluded our team of professionals.

The doctors were suspicious, however. No fever and no white count and no improvement with a full marinade of antibiotics? Something had to be wrong here. The costs were mounting. Consultants in infectious disease and oral surgery were brought in. Luckily, one of the physicians had recalled a similar patient that was presented at a regional meeting. *Nothing beats good communication.*

So as Ariel waited, the physicians continued to meet. Her white count never got higher. Her temperature never spiked. Soon her antibiotics were stopped and yet nothing changed. The doctors decided to become detectives and find out a little bit more about this patient from other hospitals she had frequented.

As luck would have it, the information started to pour in. Ariel had episodes of spontaneous pneumothoraces which required multiple operations for thoracotomies in the past. Constant admissions of subcutaneous emphysema (air under the skin) was her calling card. She claimed she would get air in her neck and chest even after a bout of sneezing. *Talk about your allergies!* When confronted by another hospital about needle marks under her left breast, poor Ariel ran away. Ariel was not gone for long though because other "incidents" would bring her in. A car accident revealed nothing major that needed hospitalization, so seven days later she shot herself in the chest. Some people really seem to like hospital food. The good news was that her wounds healed well enough from the gunshot so that she could be discharged only to be subsequently readmitted three weeks later for abscess of her chest. Again, air was found under the skin of her left chest and incision and drainage was performed. This occurred many more times for Ariel. Sometimes air would be under her neck, under her armpit, or under her breast. Sometimes her whole lung would collapse.

On one crummy day for Ariel, the staff noticed her syringe tucked away nicely in her sock. This put Ariel in a terrible mood and she felt she had to leave the hospital when she was accused of self-abusive behavior. *"How dare they question me?"* she must have thought.

Our story continues with our local heroes reading the old records and deciding to confront Ariel themselves. With one motion, she pulled out her tracheostomy tube (*Ouch!*) and left the hospital against medical advice. Attempts to follow-up with her were useless. Ariel was gone and off to see the rest of the thousands of hospitals on her schedule.

The moral of this story: think twice when seeing a patient whose skin is so bubbly you want to pop it like those wrappers used to cushion packages.✚

Adapted from the Ear, Nose & Throat Journal. *June 1998.*

THE RESIDENT

INTRODUCTION

Let me first get this out of the way – residency sucks. It was the absolute hardest thing I ever had to do in my life. *And I only did three years of it!* Neurosurgeons spend seven years after medical school, most of it on-call, finishing up their residency. This is why they make the big bucks and why I think they deserve it.

When men and women graduate medical school they finally become real doctors. Prescriptions that they write for patients actually work without the need for someone else to co-sign for them. Patients called them "doctor" even when they were medical students, but now the residents don't have to correct them. They now have more power in the treatment of the human species than they ever had before. Unfortunately, all this glory gets diminished because of how extremely overwhelmed and overworked they are. Combine that with their inexperience and you have the perfect recipe for disaster.

Residents, in general, are not happy. There tends to be a pervasive unpleasantness about them. The main reason for this is probably the long hours they work. Putting in 80 to 100 hours a week is nothing unusual for these young doctors. In fact, the medical system in our country would be even more bankrupt if it didn't survive off the backs of these underpaid workers. Residents only get paid about $20,000 to $25,000 per year, which explains a lot of their bitterness. I mean, you do the math: 80 hours a week, 50 weeks a year – *it's $6.25 an hour.* And along with poverty, pressure, and paper-work, they invariably get the toughest patients to deal with in the toughest urban areas of our country. As you can imagine, this sets up our young doctors for some incredible experiences; some are weird, others are gross, but an overwhelming number are absurdly funny.

But it's not like they come out of this unscathed: The residents suffer personal consequences of all this hard work as well. A lot of them start losing their hair. Hygiene becomes a low priority for all of them. The hierarchy of command by the more experienced doctors can be tortuous for the younger ones. Like the military, each resident has the authority to boss around the younger ones under his or her command. *In other words, shit rolls downhill and so do the grossest and worst parts of the job.* They thought medical school was tiring, but as residents their fatigue is now at an all-time high. Even though they rarely sleep and are always on the move, they still end up gaining a lot of weight. Some doctors suspect that the real reason the hospital gives them scrubs to wear is to hide their growing waistlines. There are multiple contributing factors in all this weight gain – open access to the high caloric cafeteria, free meals from pharmaceutical representatives, and the constant temptation to scam food off patients' plates. *Not that any of this food is good, mind you.* I remember that in Texas, where I trained, every table had a bottle of hot sauce on it to mask the horrible taste. They even served ox tails (cow vertebrae) at breakfast! I remember the looks I got when I asked the cafeteria workers for a dinner roll.

"We don't serve rolls at breakfast. Are you crazy?" they asked.

"But you serve freakin' ox tails?" I responded.

"You need to leave the line, sir."

Residents have other issues to deal with as well. Much of it has to do with all the time that is spent in the prison . . . *I mean the hospital.* Too many of the residents lose their sense of reality and many end up losing their families. Marriages break up. There are those affairs that arise between residents or with other hospital staff. Many residents start fighting with one another over who covers which patients or who is doing enough work. Just as everywhere else in life, there are always those slack-asses who are great at gaming the system and scamming their way out of responsibility. The other residents hate them and this only makes for more conflict and worse working conditions.

When it is all said and done, however, the resident just wants to make it through so he or she can start a real job. They look forward to finally getting paid what they are worth. They look forward to repairing relationships with their loved ones. They look forward to starting over in a fresh environment. What is funny is that, years later, physicians always look back at residency as one of the most exciting times in their lives. They can recall 20-year-old outrageous encounters with patients like they happened yesterday. Instead of being scarred for life they got through some extremely trying times and lived to boast about it. It is these stories that help define them as doctors and storytellers.

Telling a good tale enables the rest of us not only to laugh, but to be better doctors. We are proud that we were able to pry out some of the best of those anecdotes and put them here. ✚

TIMING IS EVERYTHING

I was a medical intern in Delaware and was doing my two elective months of surgery. Two surgical interns were on each night; in this case it was me and my good friend Andy B. Each night we'd finish our rounds at about 11 p.m., knock off at midnight and be up by 6 a.m. for rounds the next morning. We'd share a call room and each guy would take three hours of call. We would choose either the first or second shift, which was midnight to 3 a.m. or 3 a.m. to 6 a.m. In this way, we were pretty much guaranteed at least three or four hours of sleep if we were lucky enough to pick it right.

One night at about 11 p.m., I was walking through the halls when I saw two emergency room residents walking toward me in deep conversation. I sort of halfheartedly overheard one of them saying,

". . . and you should have seen the guy in Room 3. I mean, they found him lying in a pool of his own feces, both legs covered from top to bottom with maggots!"

His companion asked what he was going to do. The other resident replied,

"I don't know, guess I'll call surgery."

Being a medical intern, the impact of this didn't entirely register for about 10 minutes when suddenly it hit me –

I WAS SURGERY!

This now had me worried because debriding a load of maggots wasn't exactly a skill I was anxious to hone. So when Andy and I prepared to split up for the night, I'd done some figuring and made my best guess, knowing the usual efficiency of the ER.

Andy asked whether I wanted first or second shift and I replied I'd take calls from midnight to 3 a.m.

We knocked off at 11 p.m. or so and I fell into a deep sleep. I slept through my shift, luckily without any calls.

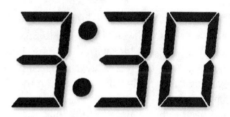

Sure enough, about 3:30 a.m. the beeper goes off and I hear Andy knock the phone off the stand and then groggily greet the ER.

"Yeah, this is Dr. B. Ummhmm. Yeah.
COVERED WITH WHAT??!!!"

Muttering and cursing, he gets up, grabs his lab coat, and disappears. I could barely keep from laughing. Next morning at rounds Andy regaled us with the details of this patient which I appreciated with mock surprise and total horror (a poker face is always important).

Five years later when we both completed our training I finally confessed. There are a lot of important issues to learn in your training to become an astute physician. None, however, is as important as being or not being at the right place at the right time. For all those residents reading this, take heed. Timing is everything in medicine. ✚

DRINKING BUDDIES

Turn the page upside down and get a whole new perspective!

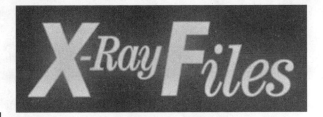

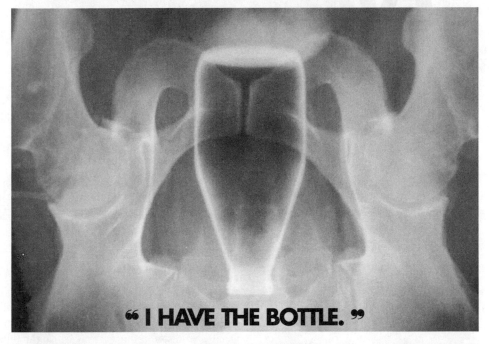

" I HAVE THE BOTTLE. "

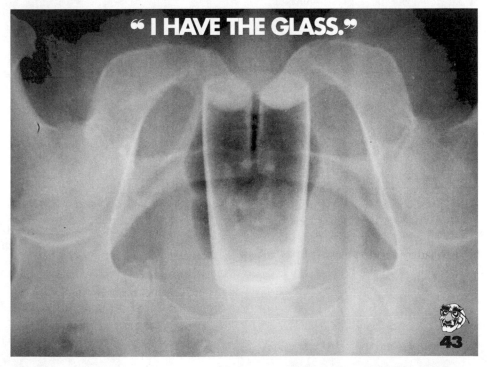

" I HAVE THE GLASS."

43

I remember it like it was yesterday.

I was on my "nights" rotation and was only an intern. They had paired me up with a second-year resident, Mike, who was known to be a little earthy, crunchy, and way too relaxed. At our residency, we didn't have call on our Internal Medicine rotation except for 36-hour stints every few weekends. Instead, we rotated through for a week of nights that started on Monday and ended on Friday morning. The two residents would come in at 5:30 p.m., stay up and work all night, and then leave the next day at 8 a.m.

this guy is a goner. He already had bacteria seen in his blood on first look by the lab. Anybody who is febrile with a dropping blood pressure and blood that looks like bacteria soup has a mortality rate near 100 percent. We explained that to his sister and her husband and we all came up with the conclusion that comfort care would be the most humane plan. Humane to Mr. Bell and humane to Mike and me, who could sprint back to bed for 20 minutes of shut-eye after minimal work.

Putting this guy in the unit for sepsis would cost thousands of dollars to the taxpayers and even worse, keep our asses up all night with phone calls from brutal and tortuous unit nurses. We all decided that comfort care would include no IV lines (and therefore no antibiotics or fluid).

AN INTERN GETS MORE

NIGHT

We received Mr. Bell on a Monday night.

It was actually going into Tuesday morning and the ER called and stated that this unassigned patient needed to be admitted. After failing in trying to block this admission with every excuse possible, Mike and I went down to put him in.

He was in his nineties and severely demented.

He lived at the Alzheimer's unit of the local psychiatric hospital and was septic. He was febrile and had severely low blood pressure. His baseline mental status was that of a wine cork. Talking to his caregivers at the other hospital showed that he was noncommunicative, did very few activities of daily living (except sit and feed himself), and had no memory of his family. We knew this because I called and talked to his sister. She was in her late eighties and actually came into the hospital with her husband. She told me that her brother had had no idea who she was for many years.

My senior resident and I had a pow-wow and came up with a plan. We figured that

We would transfer him to PO3 (a regular medical floor), which was affectionately called the "Killing Fields" only because patients with comfort care usually were sent there. Okay, because the nurses there were old psychiatric nurses and they didn't have a clue how to do much more than crochet at night.

Mr. Bell was transferred to PO3 and I beat Mike on our sprint to the other side of the hospital where I long-jumped into my bed. I did get a few minutes of sleep that night but stopped in on PO3 to see if Mr. Bell had already expired. I needed to update the new team that was to pick him up. I passed his room and he was lying in bed and not moving. No oxygen. No IV fluid or antibiotics. Nothing at all . . .

. . . but he was still breathing.

That night when I came on, the resident in charge of his care stated that Mr. Bell was still alive. Mike and I wondered how the hell this could be. How long can someone live without any fluid much less being septic?

I worked hard that night and forgot all about him. Tuesday was moving into Wednesday and I realized that morning that I had not received the death call yet.

I went over to PO3 and looked to see if a chart was still outside the room (signifying that they cleaned out the room if it wasn't). To my disbelief the chart was there and so was Mr. Bell. Thirty-six hours with no fluid and infested with blood-borne pathogens and this guy looked like a Yogi in deep meditation.

I didn't know if he was still febrile because we cancelled all vital sign checks. The nurses there loved when we minimized their work.

This is when the dreams began. Nightmares actually.

As I slept during the day at home, which wasn't easy to do comfortably, I dreamed that Mr. Bell was asking for water. It was killing me.

We then started to joke (all the day residents on Internal Medicine, Mike, and myself).

Should we leave some food or water next to his bed? Milk and cookies, like you do for Santa? Should we start antibiotics or food or pound him with a megadose of morphine? Soon the nurses asked me the same question. I jokingly said that if this guy gets up and asks for a drink, give it to him.

My last night was a bitch, but I made it through the week. I went to PO3 to see my old friend and say goodbye. Of course the damn chart with his name was still outside the door. Over 100 hours without fluid and he was still alive.

As I turned to walk in his room, I realized things had taken a turn for the worse. There was

THAN JUST BAD DREAMS

MARES

When was he going to kick off?

I truly believe we did the best thing. Even his sister said that he didn't want to live this way . . . being demented.

When I returned Wednesday night, I found out that Mr. Bell was still alive. *This guy was torturing me!* Mike and I debated again how long one can live without water. We found out that he did receive one shot of Rocephin in the ER prior to admission. I recommend we all get a shot of Rocephin when we are about to die. Seemed to have been ambrosia to Mr. Bell.

Wednesday night moved into Thursday morning and again I visited my old friend.

There was this motherfu%#&%, lying in a trance, but alive and breathing.

My rotation had one more day.

The nightmares continued.

"Water? Just a sip of water?" Now I was starting to stress. I was caught between guilt and anger. On one side I questioned my decision and on the other side I was ready to kill this bastard myself. Off I went to the last night on call. I didn't even ask if Mr. Bell was still alive. He was.

Mr. Bell sitting up with the morning breakfast platter on his lap, sipping a small glass of OJ. I didn't give him time to turn and look at me as I didn't want any more nightmares.

As far as I know, Mr. Bell is still alive today.

Like the movie *Highlander*, he may never die. I say this because someone who reads this story may someday take over his care. For that person, I recommend fresh squeezed orange juice with a slice of buttered toast. Just the way he likes it. ✛

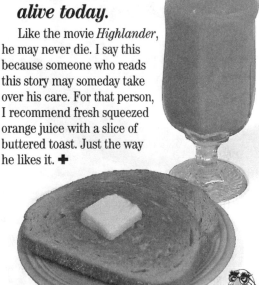

PUZZLING

As a third-year family practice resident, I started as chief of the medical service at our local community hospital. One of my patients was a middle-aged gentleman who was in for puzzling chest and upper abdominal pains. The previous team and their attendings, despite a battery of tests, were unable to ascertain the source of his pain.

Well, I sauntered in to work with him feeling, as a senior resident, that I could solve this man's problem. I did solve it, but in an unexpected way.

I did my complete history and was finishing up my physical with the mandatory rectal exam that every good house officer must do.

Suddenly the door flew open and nurses, residents, and a code cart burst on the scene.

When I asked what the heck was going on, I was told that at the moment I was performing the rectal, his monitor tracing suddenly registered 4 mm of ST depression! ***He was having a heart attack.*** Case solved. ✚

"GET ME OUT OF HERE!"

I was in the last couple of months of my internship at a county hospital in Texas. I hated that hospital and those ringing bells on all the floors which would drive anyone mad. One day I got off the elevator and turned the corner to see a handful of visitors briskly walking away from a man who was very quickly approaching me. He was a patient and seemed to have just disconnected his chest tube. There he was holding it in his hand and this thing is sucking air and gurgling.

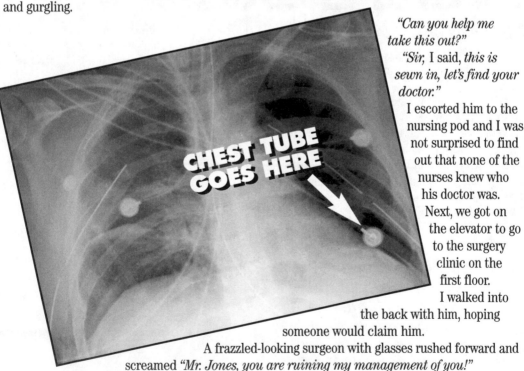

CHEST TUBE GOES HERE

"Can you help me take this out?"

"Sir, I said, *this is sewn in, let's find your doctor."*

I escorted him to the nursing pod and I was not surprised to find out that none of the nurses knew who his doctor was. Next, we got on the elevator to go to the surgery clinic on the first floor.

I walked into the back with him, hoping someone would claim him.

A frazzled-looking surgeon with glasses rushed forward and screamed *"Mr. Jones, you are ruining my management of you!"*

Mr. Jones' reply . . . *"* ***Big whoop.*** *"* ✚

EDITOR'S NOTE: Maybe we should treat patients as people and not as diseases.

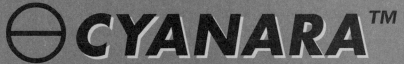
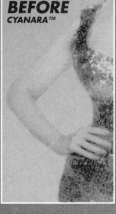
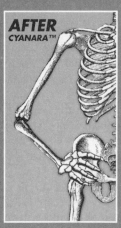

Armed and Dangerous!

Mr. Jayner was not a very complicated 38-year-old new patient. He supposedly had bipolar disorder (like who doesn't) and had come to me for back pain. A neurosurgeon gave him a discectomy nine months earlier, but he still had pain (*now that was a big surprise*). Two motor vehicle accidents later and this guy decides that I was to be his new source of pain meds.

I didn't know him from Adam, but since the neurosurgeon wouldn't give him his drugs anymore, I was to feel lucky that he was at my doorstep. That same surgeon had referred him to a physiatrist but it "didn't work out" according to the patient. After thoroughly degrading the physiatrist in front of me and calling him a quack, Mr. Jayner innocently mentions that only hydrocodone and OxyContin work for him. It must be hard for some people, with so many great medications on the market, to have your choices narrowed down to two.

I left the room and called a doctor he had seen before. He informed me that Mr. Jayner had just come out of jail and was not to be trusted. In fact, he had been abusive to his staff and they would not deal with him anymore.

When I examined him I found his acting ability quite good, but his findings quite benign. I gave him my talk about narcotics and abuse and said he didn't need this type of medicine. Funny thing, he didn't take it very well and gave me the line that we all hear, *"Then what am I supposed to do for my pain."* I offered the usual assortment of NSAIDS, but he laughed that off. Fortunately, I was able to free myself of Mr. Jayner and get him out the door, but not before he gave me lots of guilt, as well as mild threats.

Within two days he was calling our office and cursing out my receptionist. As our usual practice, we told him that we do not tolerate this type of behavior and therefore we would not deal with him anymore. He continued to make his empty threats until we hung up.

I never heard directly from Mr. Jayner

THOSE DARN NARC SEEKERS

again. An operative note from another neurosurgeon in town showed that months later he had surgery once more and then he was sent home on painkillers. Follow-up notes showed that he was doing "beautifully." I actually felt bad. It seems that I misunderstood this guy's pain and misjudged him. I guess sometimes we need to be a little more understanding of people, no matter what their past issues are, even if all the red flags of narcotic abuse are flying mightily in the wind.

Seven months later, a DEA agent and a United States Marshal showed up at our door looking for his records. I was off that day but called as soon as I could. It seems that good old Mr. Jayner does indeed have a little problem with narcotic abuse. He was recently bugging the ER for meds and when they refused and told him to leave, the police were needed to calm him down and subsequently arrest him. There also was this slight problem of anger control. In fact, Mr. Jayner was now on the loose again and was wanted for the shooting of a patrol officer. Luckily the bullet missed the cop's head by two inches and ended up plugging his patrol hat instead. The hat flew off like one of those cheap special effects you see in those old Western movies.

Anyway, Mr. Jayner didn't seem to get the rehabilitation he needed and had come out of jail to cause more problems – one of them being bothering me for narcotics. The other issues include alcohol abuse and domestic violence. He was now on the lam. The cops just wanted to know if I had seen him and warn me to be wary, as he could be armed and dangerous. They left me with a warm, loving feeling inside which proves that I am always at risk on this job. So, as I now leave this office and walk alone in the darkness to my car, I feel good that Mr. Jayner could be right around the corner looking for someone else to shoot. The NRA may recommend having small arms on my person, but I would have to refute that. A bullet wouldn't be able to stop Mr. Jayner. Pockets full of narcotics, on the other hand, would be like feeding candy to a baby. *Beat that Mr. Heston!* ✚

Lilith was a 38-year-old female with a terrible problem. *She kept getting bladder stones!*

Prior to coming to our heroes, Lilith was admitted four other times for the same thing. The first time she came in, two stones were found on the X-ray (the size of very large grapes). The second time there was only one bladder stone, but it too was large. A few months later another grape-sized stone was spotted and wouldn't you know it, there were two more located seven weeks later. Each time Lilith would have to endure a painful procedure for her recurrent lithiasis. A suprapubic cystolithotomy was the method of choice and thankfully it got the job done. Lilith braved each operation with good will and cheer, only to have the problem pop up again in the near future. *Were these physicians missing something?* The answer is yes and no.

Lilith came in for the fifth time four months later. The doctors were puzzled. Urine cultures were done but came back normal. Cystograms showed a normal urinary tract. Even an endocrine consultant gave no clue as to what was going on. Analysis of the stones showed them to be made of calcium carbonate. *What the heck was going on here?*

JUST A STONE'S THROW AWAY

Then it hit them – our authors had the brilliant hypothesis that stones this big would have ripped up (or at least dilated) the uterus on their way down from the kidneys. And this was not the case with Lilith.

Lilith was married but childless after nine years of trying. When confronted, our little sterile Munchausen denied everything. When pressed further, however, Lilith confessed that she was putting the stones into her bladder through her urethra *(Ouch!)* but she only did it because of problems with her husband and their inability to conceive. Some would say counseling or fertility pills would have worked better.

To give Lilith the credit she deserves, she was the first person ever recorded in medical research to actually put stones up her … well, you know. Secondly, a two-year follow up with Lilith showed that she had given up her little hobby. *Good job Lilith!*

Before we end, I am sure you are asking, *"Where did Lilith get her stones from?"* Good question. Analysis showed that Lilith's stones were the same as those found on the bottom of a local river. *Think of that the next time you are skipping them across the water.* ✚

The above is all TRUE but sarcastically and liberally embellished from: Acta Urologica Belgica *1998, 66, 4, 33-35.*

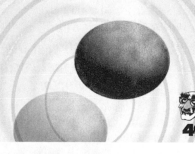

CHUX

My story begins when I was a second-year resident in family practice. I was training at a large tertiary care hospital that was located rurally. I lived out of the way in a small town of about 1,500 people and became known as "Doc" by all the locals. I was confused when my neighbor walked up to me one day and told me she saw my picture in the "paypah." Later I found out that my picture was placed in the newspaper by my residency to acquaint the residents to the community. I enjoyed the rural lifestyle, which required self-reliance, while I also worked as a medical resident continually operating out of my comfort zone on a daily basis. To be honest, I mostly enjoyed my time off, which included playing golf, skiing, and hiking every chance I got.

The following events started when my best friend from high school was visiting one fateful Saturday. He was here on his annual fishing trip, which included a couple rounds of golf followed by a long ride to a remote fishing camp that can only be accessed by boat. Basically, once you make it to the fishing camp you are stuck there for at least a week. His base camp had only generator power, which meant that it was lights out by 10 p.m. He would have only one pay phone at his disposal, but the reception was extremely poor. In other words, when Bill got to his destination there was no one there to help him.

Bill and I were finishing up our second round of golf when he stated that he felt nauseous and had been having some pain and pressure in the perineal region. I tried my best to ignore his symptoms (and not laugh too much).

Why is it that people feel they can tell you anything just because you're a doctor?

50 I encouraged him to have another beer to see if that might help his pain. He laughed and proceeded to drink several cold ones without much effect except, to my expense, tremendous bloating and flatulence. The last part actually brought tears to my eyes to the point I thought he might have something infectious in his colon – possibly fungal.

We had supper that evening and Bill became more nauseous and uncomfortable as the evening progressed. He then revealed to me that he does in fact have a long history of festering boils that come and go and tend to manifest in the groin, axilla, and posterior auricular regions. He has seen a surgeon multiple times for incision and drainage and it sounded as though Bill might have hidradenitis suppurativa. I went to bed that evening without difficulty, amazing even myself at how quickly I could forget someone else's discomfort.

Damn, I was becoming a doctor!

Bill awoke Sunday morning looking ill and felt he could not eat breakfast. He said "The pain and pressure feeling has gotten significantly worse and I now feel a bulge under my sac!" I realized at this point that I could no longer ignore my friend in need. I also thought how interesting it is the way patients describe their anatomy, especially the scrotum.

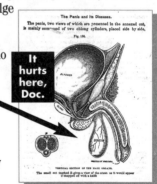

It hurts here, Doc.

Bill's annual fishing trip would certainly be ruined without some sort of immediate intervention. My advice was for Bill to mosey on up to the local ER for evaluation and treatment. However, since he had no health insurance and the possibility of hospital admission would put the kibosh on his fly-fishing trip, the answer was simple. I, the young resident in training and this man's best friend, was going to have to take control of this situation and either fix him up or possibly f%ck him up.

As we all know, a little knowledge is a dangerous thing. I was contemplating how I had just enough knowledge to be lethal when I decided to examine my best friend of over twenty years. **It's one thing to ask a total stranger to drop 'em and bend over, but it's another totally disgusting thing to ask a middle-aged friend who is semi-toxic from alcohol and bacteria to assume "the position."**

We found a quiet place and Bill bared his generous, sweaty, infected bottom to my semi-trained eyes.

Yes, there definitely was problem here. I was almost sure of it.

Bill had a large, swollen, shiny, tender erythematous mass covering his entire perineum. It was not clear at first if this was a scrotal hernia gone south, a femoral artery aneurysm ready to blow, a perirectal abscess with vigor, a tumor, or maybe just an alien. With considerable deliberation I decided that this was likely an abscess – or maybe the alien.

I had several flashbacks come to me from those surgical lectures I had in med school. Our instructor was a crusty, weathered old surgeon who always will be remembered for his unique approach to dealing with abscesses. His rules were "Never let the sun go down on an abscess" and "When you cut one open, be sure to cut a hole big enough for a prairie dog to jump through." And of course, "Cold steel cures."

It was time to move, so Bill and I made the drive into the clinic at the hospital. Being Sunday it was luckily closed and no one was around to get me in trouble for treating a patient on the side. The problem was that when we snuck into the procedure room, we found all the surgical instruments, including anesthetics, drapes, gauze, and packing were locked up tight. I went to my cubicle and found a sterile #11 blade as well as some betadine, 4 x 4's and sterile dressing. I had Bill assume the position once more and explained everything to him this way: *"I have some good news and some bad news. The good news is that I have located enough sterile equipment to get the job done. The bad news is that I don't have any topical anesthetic to apply to the area!"*

He groaned and stated that he didn't give a rat's ass! He also mentioned to

Hurry the fu#k up!

With this reassurance, I quickly prepped the area and found some **CHUX** (absorbent medical pads) for the mess. Without hesitation (okay, a lot of hesitation), I carefully made a linear incision "big enough for a prairie dog" along the long axis of this enormous abscess.

Immediately I jumped back. *Wow!* Right up side my head I was hit with the foulest smell I can ever remember. It seemed to be a cross between vomit, necrotic tissue, and toe jam.

Instantly a river of pus began to run out of this thing. The two **CHUX** were quickly overwhelmed with smelly custard and blood-colored nastiness. Within the pus, there were occasional islands or boats of solid funk floating out onto the floor across the edge of the **CHUX**.

Bill had immediate relief of his pain and in fact, he seemed to be almost orgasmic. Here I am turning blue and this guy was euphoric on some kind of sadomasochistic acid trip. His pain was gone and his nausea subsided shortly thereafter.

Bill went on his remote fishing trip without incident. I spent the rest of the day cleaning my sneakers. Bill loves to tell this story at family gatherings and parties and I squirm a little when he does. I think about being a resident and how medical training demands that you operate out of your comfort zone on a daily basis – and do it without error.

I also think about the strange relationship doctors have with their families and friends. On one hand, we are asked medical questions and opinions regularly, which the family (usually my wife) will either embrace or ignore depending on their own perceived diagnosis, prognosis, or whim. I think most physicians cringe at the thought of the saying . . .

"Is there a doctor in the house?"

I suppose this is the cross we bear for the rights and the responsibilities of our profession. There may never be a limit to this role, but if there ever was one, it would be dealing with an angry-looking rectum with a bulging abscess – or an alien. ✚

A Sticky Situation

After finishing medical school, I still wasn't sure what I wanted to do. I had a number of relatives who were surgeons and thought this might be a good area of specialization for me. Fortunately, I was able to get a rotating internship in a large city hospital in the East where I could concentrate on the surgical specialties.

During my general surgery rotation I worked the usual long hours with little sleep and poor eating habits, which was the norm in those days.

We had a patient, Lester,

who had a long-standing ulcer of the stomach with frequent vomiting which was due to a complete obstruction. Despite his malnourished state, our hands were forced and he had to have a 90 percent gastrectomy by our very aggressive third-year surgical resident.

As an intern on service, I got to spend long hours with Lester pre-op and post-op. Following surgery,

he didn't do much better in the vomiting department

and this didn't help with his incision's healing. In fact, late every afternoon, the unfortunate fellow would have vigorous emesis which resulted in daily wound dehiscence during the first post-op week. We maintained Lester on needed transfusions and IV fluids, but he eventually "ran out of veins" and we had just one remaining site,

his right jugular vein in his neck.

Unfortunately the need for a new IV site occurred right at supper time. I was getting hypoglycemic so I popped a couple of sticks of Juicy Fruit gum into my mouth and got the patient ready for the procedure. Since this was an emergency, Lester had to have his neck "cut down" at the bedside.

I made the incision and started to carefully dissect for that "last vein." The resident (*did I mention he was very aggressive*) couldn't stand to wait so he took over pretty quickly.

How's that for instilling confidence in your intern?

At this point things got really tense. The vein was very tiny and we both were concentrating very hard not to lose it. The first couple of ties slipped off. The light was poor and it was stuffy on the ward and we were both sweating up a storm. As I opened up my mouth to say something encouraging,

the piece of Juicy Fruit fell right into the incision.

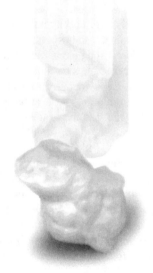

The angry resident made only one comment, *"Get that Goddamned thing out of there!!!!"*

I could not have been more embarrassed. Luckily things turned out all right for everybody. Lester recovered and was discharged after a long stay with us. I rethought my choice of specialties and decided that my Juicy Fruit and I might be better attuned to Internal Medicine.

As for the very aggressive resident

. . . actually, who cares?

✚

52

It was the first day of my surgical residency in a large Midwestern hospital. I started on the trauma service which was a grueling rotation. As luck would have it, I was on-call the first night. *I couldn't wait to get started.* Literally, I couldn't wait because before we could even finish morning rounds, the calls started to come in.

The first patient had ascending cholangitis and went into respiratory arrest. The crash cart was summoned and the second-year surgical resident adeptly inserted an endotracheal tube into the patient's lungs. As I watched, I saw the patient cough up a large, yellowish-green mucous honker which hung so grotesquely from the ET tube that I wanted to puke.

"Where's the ambu bag?" the resident asked the nurse. The nurse who had brought the crash cart couldn't find one. *"Isn't someone going to ventilate the patient?"* she asked as she glanced at me with an attitude. Shielding my incompetence (and not letting an intern do something stupid), the second-year resident replied "You ventilate the patient" to the nurse. With that she grasped the gravity of the situation and ran from the patient's room to find an ambu bag. The rest of us left to go on rounds except the second-year resident, who stayed to enjoy his time with the patient (and the nurse).

This was going to be fun, I thought. By the time we reached the stairwell to move onto the next floor, seven pagers went off at once like something out of a Sci-Fi movie.

"Trauma Alert. Trauma Alert. Three minutes."

It was surreal and the whole progression stopped in its tracks. The beauty was that I had no idea what a trauma alert was. It is a good thing they gave me the responsibility of holding on to the pager.

With a blink of an eye, most of the group whisked off to the ER to treat the first of many stabbing victims that would come in that day. I was one of the few left to finish rounds. One by one our group was being "picked off" and I was praying all along not to be left alone. Fortunately, it didn't happen.

The day continued with a *treat* from our senior resident. He wanted to look in on an autopsy of a patient who had died from necrotizing fasciitis.

The "flesh-eating" bacteria pervaded the room with such a stench that it was almost unbearable. I've known some bad smells but this was the worst. *As an intern, you are at the senior resident's whim.* As he chatted with his buddy, the pathologist, I was trapped there breathing in death.

A little later, the pagers started up again. The first one was an ENT (Ear, Nose, and Throat) resident wanting me to come to the recovery room to put chest tubes in one of his patients. The guy had bilateral tension pneumothoraces after his tracheostomy. *Remind me never to have a tracheostomy July 1st at a teaching hospital.* By the time I told him it was my first day he was already paging the third-year resident. I went to see how things were going and the third-year was already there with tubes in place. He directed me to the radiographic viewbox to see the most collapsed lung nubbins I had ever seen *(actually, I had never seen any)*.

Thank goodness he was there to help or else this patient would have been left with me. My chance to shine that day came with a nursing home patient who had a fever and abdominal pain. On rounds, the senior resident wanted me to do the rectal exam after everyone left. Sure enough, the lady had a rectal mass. *I was a hero.*

I waited until the afternoon rounds to disclose my findings. I told the group that I had felt rectal cancer before *(bluffing)*, but this was different. It was rock hard, but smooth and oddly shaped. We moved on and the senior resident came back with me to do a complete pelvic exam. Our patient didn't have rectal cancer but a foul-smelling pessary that had eroded through the vaginal wall. I was humbled. *I didn't even know what a pessary was. Now I do, and it's not cancer.*

My first day concluded with my feet killing me and my pride hurting even worse. I am sure I wasn't the first to go through this initiation or trial by fire. It still didn't make it any easier. I am wiser now. I am more experienced now. As I sit back and write about trauma, chest tubes, smells and pessaries I realize how glad I am to be done with it all and laugh because I know some schmuck somewhere is now going through the same thing. ✚

53

FIRST

My story begins as an intern at a large teaching hospital. The internal medicine teaching service was our toughest rotation. During the daytime the house staff included a senior resident, junior residents, two or three interns, and several Medicine attendings. The residents rounded in the early morning hours and had formal sit down rounds at 10 a.m. The nights were covered by a senior and a junior resident who worked block nights, this consisted of 100-hour weeks, six nights a week, with Sundays off to lick your wounds and dry out your crying towel.

Cases admitted overnight (known as hits) were presented at sit-down rounds the next morning complete with EKGs, X-rays, labs, etc. This was the resident's chance to sink or swim and the senior resident rarely presented cases at rounds (*they paid their dues as an intern*). The attendings seemed to enjoy sit-down rounds, it was their chance to drink coffee, discuss fascinating medical cases, and conduct their own twisted version of *The Weakest Link* with the housestaff. After taking your licks at rounds, the night crew would stagger home, depressed from sleep deprivation, exhaustion, ego assassination, and bad hair. They would then try to get some sleep with the sun beaming in their window, only to be woken up by the friggin' alarm and begin their night all over again (like a bad Groundhog Day movie). Frequently the night crew fought with one another as well as with the nurses, other residents, ER attendings, RNs, and our own attendings who don't want to get out of bed in the middle of the night (*remember, they paid their dues too*).

TRADITION IS A FUNNY THING.
Tradition is alive and well in academic medicine.
All of us agree that overworked, depressed, and borderline psychotic interns are a danger to themselves and all patients with whom they come in contact. On the other hand . . . *few of us want to see these*

interns skate through their internship and residency without the pain, hardship, and emotional scars that all physicians endure in training. The wounds run deep and are quickly opened up even 20 or 30 years later. No physician should escape that horror, all must run the gauntlet (*flashback to the movie* Apocalypse Now *where Marlon Brando discusses "The horror, the horror" shortly before his death*).

The case that sticks out in my mind occurred on my **FIRST NIGHT** of Medicine rotation in my internship year. I was excited and somewhat nervous about starting the night shift. It was billed as a tremendous learning experience and a chance to fly solo, run some codes, and practice real medicine. I was teamed up with Sandy, a third-year resident who was very bright and upbeat. I considered myself lucky to be working with Sandy since I had lots to learn. We were getting coffee when the beeper went off. Something about a "GI bleeder" was all Sandy said. *I was pumped! A real medicine case!* Not some "namby pamby" 90-year-old dehydrated, demented, incontinent nursing home horror show who was sent over so her covering nurse could have some respite. The ER doctor gave us the bullet presentation and did the ceremonious passing of the chart to me (*it was like handing over the keys to a car that was on fire*). "Her pressure is kind of soft and her labs aren't back yet." My naiveté was suddenly exposed as I watched the senior resident's eyebrows twitch at the word "soft."

Our patient was in the critical care section of the ER. She was sitting on her gurney, all 275 pounds of her. She was inebriated, reeking of alcohol, the NG (nasogastric) tube was stuck in her nose and her face and mouth were covered with charcoal. *A very pretty picture.* She was a suspected polysubstance abuser and subsequently now had a GI bleed. She was a frequent flyer and the ER staff was on a first-name basis with her and knew her life story (with intimate details).

NIGHT

A NIGHT I WOULD RATHER FORGET

As I approached the gurney Sandy threw a yellow smock, a face shield, and gloves at me. *"Put these on . . . you'll need 'em."* I interviewed the patient after reviewing her previous 12 charts in the ER. I learned nothing new from the interview with the patient that was not already well documented in her history except for the two things she said to me, *"You suck"* and *"I'm leaving."*

Her labs starting coming back and we found out that her alcohol levels were high and her blood counts were low. Her toxicology screens were positive for benzodiazapenes and cannabis (*"Party on Wayne, party on Garth"*). Just as the nurse was handing me a fresh set of vital signs, both our code beepers went off. Sandy moved fast. *"It's in the ICU, I'll go . . . you stay here!"* Sounded like a good idea.

As Sandy was taking off her smock and face shield the patient sat up, looked directly at Sandy and in slow motion projectile vomited one warm fresh quart of blood, alcohol, bile, and charcoal all over Sandy's face, chest, and arms. *"Motherf*cker!"* Sandy ran out of the ER to her code and did not have time to shower off her new look.

The ER nurse started yelling out numbers at me *"70 systolic over palp, what do you want to do?"* . . . **Let's see, I've never managed a GI bleed or for that matter a critical care case and I have now just sh#t me pants. Hmm, ahh, let's ahhmmm. Give blood, yes lots of blood!** *Bold move, Einstein!* The patient began to vomit bright red blood at an alarming rate; she filled a large basin on her lap. The nurses guessed about 5 to 6 liters. The experienced ER nurses started smelling panic and fear; I needed to do something substantial. What I really thought was "How else can I stall until Sandy gets back?" As quickly as the nurses pumped in the blood through two large bore needles, it came back out. I decided to call the gastroenterologist on-call. Yeah, that's if he'll help me. At 2 a.m. most attendings don't answer the pager on the first page. Twenty minutes and two pages later, I got a hold of Dr. Letmesleep on the horn. *"Yeah, that sounds bad, why don't you get the patient stable in the ICU and I'll see her –"* CLICK. **Wait a minute, need help now, please, I beg of you!** I then called the surgeon

on-call for his opinion. Again I gave my 30-second history hoping he would bite. He didn't. *"Sounds like she's going to die –"* and *"Call Gastro –"* CLICK. I felt like the "newbies" in the movie *Platoon*, going out for an all-night ambush expecting a firefight with the enemy and placing the most inexperienced, greenest soldiers at the point position – the point most likely to confront the enemy. *Why, do you ask, would they do this?*

TRADITION!

(I could just picture myself presenting this case at rounds the next morning. "You are the weakest link, good bye!") I got out my Ferris' manual and flipped to GI bleeds. The nurses began to roll their eyes; they fully understood the gravity of the situation. **By the way, nurses do hate interns. Why? Because technically an intern is a doctor, but he/she is a special kind of doctor, the kind that doesn't know squat!**

I finally realized Sandy wasn't coming back anytime soon. It looked like esophageal varices or possibly a Mallory-Weiss tear. I blurted out an order to give vasopressin using the most confident reassuring voice I could muster. I believed in my heart that the administration of this obscure medication (which I read about but never even prescribed before) would have no effect on the patient's condition. The nurses smirked and ran to get the medicine. Like magic, the medicine stopped the bleeding immediately and the patient's blood pressure rebounded.

What odds! Had I won the lottery?

How did this end? The patient lived to drink and drug another day. *Me?* After some sleep, I got pimped unmercifully at rounds the next morning on the 900 causes of upper GI bleeds. Oh yeah, the gastroenterologist who saw the bleeder the next morning in the ICU confirmed that she did in fact have esophageal varices and said, *"You might want to try octreotide next time, it's a new somatostatin analog with an improved side effect profile over vasopressin."*

Thanks for the help, assh#le! ✚

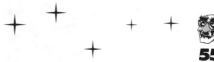

I was a fourth-year resident doing ER rotation at George Washington University in about 1984 when I picked up a Middle Eastern patient in Room 4. His history was kind of unusual. He was in renal failure and was fed up with using dialysis. Upon hearing that GW had a few good transplant surgeons of Middle Eastern background, he decided on his own to grab a jet and fly on over for his transplant. He hadn't been worked up, referred, matched, or anything. He sort of treated the situation just like going to the store. He arrived having not been dialyzed for several days. He simply came to the ER with a translator from his embassy expecting to get admitted and transplanted. This gentleman did not look very good at all. He was very weak and his skin was a combination of yellow and tan.

I was there with a nurse getting a good history and preparing to examine him when he started to vomit. This wasn't your usual vomit. This stuff was really copious, nothing was digested, and it just struck me as unusual. He'd eaten a load of linguine or something on the plane and it was so sudden and voluminous that I grabbed a bedpan to handle the load. Then . . .

smack in the middle of the emesis,

was one particular piece of linguine that was bigger, thicker, and sort of brown on the end. Even worse, it started moving about like a cobra. This, I assure you, may be fairly common in certain locales, but Foggy Bottom, DC, is not one of them. The nurse's eyes, as well as mine, were as big as saucers. The patient looked sort of bemused, but not particularly shocked.

When he finished singing lunch, I staggered out to Dr. Mark Smathers, the attending. I tried to interrupt the four phone conversations he was having at once.

"Dr. Smathers," I said. He waved me off with a hand gesture.

"Dr. Smathers!" I said with more urgency. Nothing. Finally I faced him and blurted out, ***"The patient in room four just puked up a ten-inch-long ascaris."***

He immediately put down all four phones, looked at me with equally astonished eyes, and without missing a beat, said, *"Take it up to pathology."* I used two cervical swabs like a pair of chopsticks, picked up the worm and

dropped it in a urine cup.

At that point I walked it up to pathology. There was a bored path student on work-study checking in specimens who didn't even look as I dropped off the cup. When I told him what was in it, he jumped out of his chair like I had just given him a shrunken head. Upon returning to the patient, he and his translator both had inquisitive looks on their faces. The translator said, ***"He vants to know vot heppent to de vurm."*** It almost seemed as if he was missing his close friend or something.

I thought this is one of my greatest medical stories and definitely wanted to share it. When I told it to one of the female residents in my class (sort of the med school equivalent of putting a frog in her desk in grade school), she coldly turned toward me and said, in that obnoxious voice of hers, ***"That's a quite common occurrence in areas where parasites are endemic."***

My only prayer is that someday she has a nice bowl of moving linguine made especially for her.

PASTA ANYONE

It had been a busy morning. In our Occupational Medicine Clinic we frequently see follow-up visits for lacerations. I noticed that a laceration was to be brought back as the last patient of the morning. It looked like about a week since the date of injury, and usually stitches can just be taken out and the patient sent on their way quickly. In order to speed things up and be able to have more time for lunch, I grabbed the chart, went into the waiting room and called the gentleman's name.

Hi, *"I'm Dr. Smith. So, Mr. Burke, rumor has it that you have some stitches –*

if you could let me take a quick look I'll have Dan, our medical assistant, take you back to get them out."
I looked at his hands. He replied, *"Doc, I don't think you want me to do that – they're on my scrotum."*
I felt terrible as all the staff heard the dilemma as well. I must have turned several shades of red. Thankfully, the guy was very nice – even in spite of his horrible work injury. *He had been emptying a Dumpster and slipped . . . It was a freak accident.* He did very well. However, my staff would not let me live it down – and whenever we have a laceration, I make very sure to read the chart first. ✚

OUCH!

BRIGHT LIGHTS

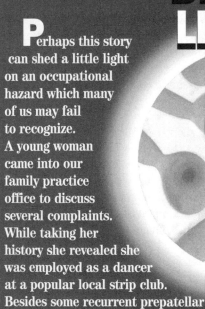

Perhaps this story can shed a little light on an occupational hazard which many of us may fail to recognize. A young woman came into our family practice office to discuss several complaints. While taking her history she revealed she was employed as a dancer at a popular local strip club. Besides some recurrent prepatellar bursitis she also complained of a vaginal discharge. Her wet prep revealed fungal elements. When she was informed, she was quite taken aback and expressed her need for an immediate cure. She explained, *"A yeast infection glows bright white under the black lights!!!! It keeps customers away!"* ✚

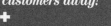

Diener

I spent some time as a pathology resident before I decided to be a "real doc." One hot, bright July, I received a page commanding that an autopsy was to be done. Autopsies and the rare frozen sections, to be looked at under the microscope, were the only pages path residents had to answer (*the good old days!*). I gathered up the diener, but couldn't find the body. A diener is some kind of German word for "helper." The dieners are the guys who do the dirty work on the autopsies while the path resident supposedly does the intellectual stuff.

It was an old medical school with multiple hospitals and morgues so we started to make the rounds. Finally we decided to look in the oldest, most unused morgue, and what do you know, there the body was! *All four hundred pounds of it on the top shelf!* I, being skinny, but confident, assured my muscular deiner that I could hold up my end, but alas, I couldn't and while trying to lower the body, *four hundred pounds of dead, cold meat hit him square and put him down!* While he was screaming under the body, I saw what would have prevented the whole mess if the light hadn't been so dim: an electric winch on the ceiling! So I buckled the winch cable under the body but got the deiner's arm in the process! After a couple more tries, the body rose up, and just as he was crawling free, I found out, unfortunately, that I had accidentally hooked the cable through another shelf holding two more bodies and tore it from the wall!

Two more bodies landed on top of my moaning deiner!

I was laughing so hard that I almost couldn't pull the bodies off of him, and, after propping them up against the wall in a sitting position, off we went to do the grossest autopsy I have ever done in my life. *Four hundred pounds of frozen lard.* ✚

Rub

Toward the end of my rotating "transitional medicine" internship, I was working in the Emergency Department. I picked up a chart for a teenage female with a chief complaint of pain with urination. In medical school, I had been told that cystitis (bladder infections) commonly occurs in women at the time when they first become sexually active. The patient was sixteen, so everything seemed to fit.

I went to the waiting room and called for the patient. Her mother came along unbidden as I lead her to the gynecology room. I introduced myself and began to ask about the history of present illness. Actually, I was stalling for time while I tried to think of a tactful way to tell the patient's mother to leave the room so that I could take an accurate sexual history. I asked relatively inane questions such as . . .

"How long have you had this pain?" and "Can you describe the pain?"

"Can you describe the pain?" elicited more than I was mentally prepared for. My attractive young patient replied by describing her symptom with the phrase, *"Well, you know how it feels when somebody rubs your clitoris too hard?"*

I don't know if my attempt to maintain a nonchalant expression was successful or not as I nodded silently. At least I knew that I no longer had to worry about how to dispense with the patient's mother, who was still sitting in the exam room with us. *Actually, being male, I have absolutely no earthly idea what having one's clitoris rubbed too hard feels like.*

The female chaperone, who was in the room with me, refused to further my medical education when I asked her about it at the nurse's station. ✚

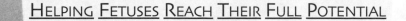

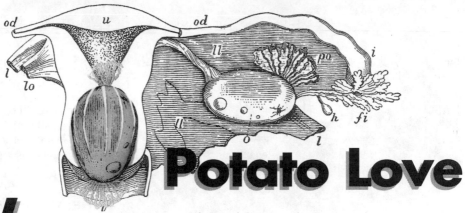

Potato Love

While doing a night shift in the ER (urban community hospital) during my family practice residency, I had the opportunity to care for a middle-aged woman whose chief complaint was *"potatoes in my pajama."* This was as close as I could get to standard English. Her speech may have been affected by the large doses of psychotropic drugs she was on. As she indicated to the nursing staff that this was a "female" problem, I found her in the pelvic room. As the history was pretty much unintelligible, I got right into the exam. There were indeed potatoes (wedges)! ***Even worse, they were sprouting inside her vagina (or in her case, in her pajama).*** Their degree of sproutedness (and other olfactory input) indicated they'd been there for some time. I of course asked her *"why did you put potatoes there?"* To paraphrase her reply, it was her method of contraception. Probably pretty damn effective too, I'll bet. ✚

EDITOR'S NOTE – Wouldn't her partner be uncomfortable with a potato? Actually, I wonder if he should just break up with the girl and have sex with the potato on its own. Seems like a lot less hassle.

A New Year

As a family practice intern, of course I was on duty for every holiday. I spent New Year's Eve on the "Labor Hall" that year. I thought, *"Hey, if you have to be on duty why not try to deliver the FIRST BABY OF THE YEAR?!"* I had lots of potential candidates and I delivered one infant at 11:30 p.m., but it wasn't close enough. Then another patient began pushing which got me excited all over again.

Now at that time, the University Hospital didn't publish the births of unwed mothers (which were a large portion of the deliveries). The next baby was born at 12:04 but to an unwed mother. We couldn't tell the world about that child, which meant I still had a chance to attain my goal. I went to the next room to deliver a woman who was also pushing and made sure that she was married.

"Oh yes," she said.

"Great!" I thought to myself, *"I've still got a shot at it."*

So I sent the husband off to change into scrubs and took the patient into the delivery room. After I draped her, I told the nurse to go get the husband and LET'S HAVE A BABY!

The patient said *"Dr. Ray, I've got to ask you something."*

"What's that ma'am?"

"Do I still get all the free stuff for the first baby of the year if the baby is not my husband's?" she asked.

The loud clunk we heard was the husband who had just entered the room doing a face plant on the floor.

The baby was delivered uneventfully, fortunately. ✚

Need a Bed

While running the FP medical service as a third-year resident at our community hospital, I had the privilege of working with many great local attendings. One morning I received a call from one of our best and busiest attendings asking me to do an admission for him. It seems that one of his chronically ill patients needed a hospital bed. I greeted the patient on his stretcher with his orderlies at the elevator door on the second floor. Surprisingly, Mr. L was kicking and screaming to the best of his frail abilities, yelling at the orderlies to let him go and that he didn't want to come in to the hospital. The orderlies were dutifully trying to calm him down . . .

"There, there, Mr. L, sir, we'll get you to your room and take good care of you." As I began my history it soon became apparent that Mr. L had indeed called his doctor's office to request help with the **purchase** of an actual hospital-style bed to use in his home to make it easier for him to be cared for there. The message as it reached his attending was interpreted as Mr. L needing hospital admission, and he got all the way to the floor before we figured this out!

Needless to say, my phone presentation to my attending was thoroughly enjoyable. ✚

NOW THAT'S A RECTAL!

I am employed as an academic attending physician in a community hospital with a residency training program in emergency medicine. One night, as I had received sign out from the day shift attending, a pleasant Latino gentleman came to triage complaining of chest pain. Mr. Sanchez, as we will call him, was whisked to a small exam room off the side of the emergency department. A tech was muttering about having to do an EKG "stat" as Mr. Sanchez stated that he had been having chest pain for more than five hours. At one point, the tech even turned to the nurse and remarked, *"Like he's really having the big one. What a waste of time."*

Well, true to form, patients will always be the wiser and he was having the proverbial "BIG ONE." The tombstones in the inferior EKG leads were pretty self-explanatory. After a cursory review of the EKG with the intern, I ordered aspirin, beta-blockers, nitrates, and thrombolytics. I asked the intern to start three IVs and do a stool guiaic (checking for blood).

As I was seated ten feet from the patient writing the orders, the intern embarked upon his tasks. The intern's name was Dr. Block and he was a gentle soul, but had a rather dominating presence, being about 6'3" and solidly built. While I'm scribbling orders and calling the cardiologist, I hear the tech shout (yes, the same one who questioned the chest pain prior to the EKG), *"Doc (me), I think you better get here. Quick!"*

As I ran to the patient's bedside I was a bit surprised to find the intern still wearing a surgi-lubricated glove with a stool specimen on the index finger and the patient now in ventricular fibrillation. **This rhythm means imminent death.** A couple hundred jolts of electricity with the defibrillator and Retavase was just what the doctor ordered.

Mr. Sanchez sailed through with flying colors but the intern to this day is still a bit leery of doing rectal examinations. It will take time for him to realize that he doesn't have the *"finger of death."* ✚

NO ⊘ SELF-DEFECATION!

I was a young intern on the internal medicine service. I had a lot to learn. I still believed everyone. *Why would some people lie?* **JOAN** was unassigned, which meant she didn't have a physician to take care of her while she was an inpatient. Her lower back **PAIN** was severe and she looked like death warmed over. I jumped in on the case with vigor and ran every obscure test known to man. Nothing came back positive to find the cause of her pain. She would cry when answers weren't found. Her husband pressed hard for someone to do something. That someone, that Hero, that fresh new doctor who was to find an answer was **me.**

She was in her thirties and was seemingly incapacitated, at least during the times that I saw her in the hospital room. She laid there getting narcotic after narcotic for a whole week. She was in so much pain that at times she defecated on herself because she couldn't get up to go to the bathroom. My buddies on the service said I was being fooled. *"She is a narc seeker. Get her out of there."* I even went to the chief of the medicine service for support and presented the case one-on-one. His response, *"Munchausen."* The only other test he could imagine getting was urine porphyrin to rule out an even more obscure disease. We were a send-out lab and it was going to take time (*it eventually came back negative*). With much prompting, I eventually was able to nudge Joan out of the hospital and back home. Of course, she did go home with a boatload of narcotics.

When she appeared the next day for readmission (*and out of narcotics*), I could have gotten someone else to cover her care. I was leaving for the night and was also finished with the medicine service. The next crew was coming on and would have taken her. But I

THOSE DARN NARC SEEKERS

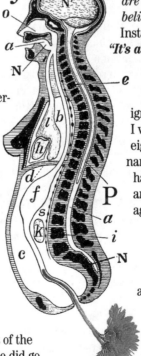

Fig. 2.—Diagrammatic longitudinal section of the Body.

was "her Hero" and her doctor. I was going to save her. I said to myself, *"Only I can take care of Joan."* I called in orders for a morphine drip and later that night went to go meet her on the floor in her room. **I was a proud man.** I felt good about myself as I walked down the long corridor to where she was. I was finally a doctor and this person needed me.

Prior to entering the room, I saw some flowers in a garbage can near the nurse's station. I picked one out and made my way in. When she saw me and saw the flower, it was too much for Joan. She burst into tears. It warmed my heart. I knew the next words were going to be something like, *"You are the best doctor"* or *"No one would believe me but you. Thank you!"* Instead, Joan began to tearfully scream, *"It's all a lie. I just wanted the drugs."*

I learned a valuable lesson that day. Forget about being the greatest doctor. It's an illusion anyway. I ignored everyone else's warning. Hell, I was blinded. She could have snorted eight pounds of OxyContin with remnants all over her face and I would have missed it. I left Joan that night and thought I never would see her again.

A year later while shopping at a local clothing outlet, I was sitting in my car waiting for my wife. Out of nowhere comes Joan and her husband walking right toward my car. She looked happy. She wasn't in any pain. **I was in pain.** Another year of residency, however, had taught me well and I was also wiser now. As she looked up at my car, I immediately did the professional thing and dove down into the passenger side to hide. My pain was better and I didn't even defecate on myself. ✚

MY FAVORITE MUNCHAUSEN

ROSEY THE RED

"Rosey" was 17 years old and very bothered by the fact she was always spitting up blood. *Wouldn't you be?* The otolaryngology clinic couldn't find a reason for her dilemma. The diagnostic tests including abdominal ultrasound, rectoscopy, esophagogastroscopy, and thoracic CT scan, were all normal. Being anemic with a slightly low hemoglobin kept everyone puzzled. The hematologic clinic thought they would get to the bottom of things, but alas, it was not to be. No local source of bleeding and no malignancy could be spotted. As the hemoglobin dropped more (below 7), five units of blood were pumped into Rosey to make her well.

All anyone could come up with was good old-fashioned iron deficiency anemia and therefore more tests were run – a good thing too. A chest X-ray, thoracic CT (repeated), and digital subtracted angiography were performed, but gave no new answers. Luckily a labeled RBC scan, two endoscopies, repeated bronchoscopies, and a partridge in a pear tree were added to the work-up. Unfortunately, they came up empty as well.

As she continued to spit up more blood, she received more transfusions. This was a nice trade off. Funny thing, no one ever actually saw Rosey spit up the blood. They just kept finding blood on her dressings. Eerily, Rosey was very blasé about the whole thing, and though it crossed the mind of the clinicians that she might be faking, they couldn't find an injection site or ecchymosis that would lead them down that road.

Was it another true mystery of science? We think not.

Interestingly enough, as they tried to discharge Rosey she would always have another "bleeding attack." Like fly paper, they couldn't dislodge themselves from this patient. Finally, one astute examiner found a scar on her elbow.

It seems Rosey had an affinity for needling herself on this part of her anatomy.

A more in-depth and less costly search showed that she coincidentally had a bloody syringe in her pants. *Some people have all the fun.*

Rosey finally fessed up to the whole charade, but blamed it all on her family problems. Maybe not getting enough toys on her birthday made her want to bloodlet herself. As far-fetched as this may sound, she never did follow up with outpatient psychotherapy.

No one knows where Rosey is today, but we at *Placebo Journal* recommend you watch your rising medical costs when rubbing elbows with this wonderful patient who could be roaming through a town like yours. ✚

Gurkan, et al. Aust NZ J Med *2000; 39.*

63

Resident physician's salaries in the early 1960s were meager at best.

DIGIT OF DEATH

Although technically illegal, supplementary income was necessary for those of us tottering under the weight of educational loans. After-hours jobs were passed on to underlings by those graduating residents leaving the Medical Center's walls for "The Real Dough," as we so crassly put it. Doing insurance physicals in Detroit's less desirable areas was a common misdemeanor, since insurance companies' physicians did not care to venture there. Actually practicing in an overburdened general practitioner's office was close to felonious.

Some sources of supplementation were ingenious. We who'd impregnated our wives were showered with baby supplies from drug companies seeking future consideration. These were immediately sold to the nurses at ten cents on the dollar. In a more visceral approach, most of us visited the blood bank every eight weeks to exchange a pint of red stuff for twenty-five dollars cash. Over my four years of specialty training, I'd sampled all these avenues of income, moving up in the hierarchy of choice each year.

As my senior residency began, I was introduced to the number-one money-maker of clandestine cash cows by the graduating Bill Johnson, M.D. The work was simple enough — twice weekly, the occupants of a nursing home on Eight Mile Road needed cursory checks to fulfill a state requirement. At fifty bucks a month, a quarter of my salary, this was a real plum.

 Rounds were between six and seven in the morning, when 20 patients were examined, vital signs taken, and medications reviewed. This time was chosen

because each morning at eight, the Operating Room schedule began. Being late for a surgical assignment was a mortal sin.

The incident occurred during my orientation visit to the nursing home. Bill was flitting around, saying goodbye to the staff. I was somewhat surprised to find the entire ambulatory population awake, quietly sitting in the reception hall, awaiting their exams. I guessed the adage of "rising early" as one ages was correct.

With farewells completed, the aged patients stared intently at "The New Doc," as we methodically did our exams. Bill was showing me the basic chart procedures when I happened to glance at a white-haired codger sitting in a corner. He looked incredibly old and incredibly awful, with a florid, almost cyanotic face, glazed eyes, and breaths coming in shallow gasps. I tapped Bill on the shoulder, pointed to the old man and said, in a voice louder than intended, *"That guy's going to die."* In retrospect, this was one of the dumber things I've done in my life. My statement was meant only as a generic opinion, but as God is my witness — *at that precise moment, the fellow exhaled a death rattle and slumped down in his wheelchair, motionless!*

Bill rushed to his side, checking for a carotid pulse. Finding none, he checked for other vital signs. Next, he beckoned to the head nurse and whispered something to her. In a few moments, an orderly arrived, who covered, then whisked the corpse from the reception hall. And during those few minutes, I saw every eye in the room upon me, and could hear a soft muttering among the clientele. Bill and I quickly finished our rounds and departed, hardly commenting on what had occurred.

Three days later, I arrived at exactly 6 a.m. for my first solo appearance. I walked in to find an empty reception hall. Nope, nary a patient to be seen. Not that there was silence, for from each of the two corridors, I could hear shouting and even a few high-pitched screams. The head nurse approached me to explain. It seems a daybreak announcement had reminded the population that "The New Doc" was coming today, and henceforth would be seeing them. The word spread like a contagion and a world-class octogenarian mutiny ensued. My imminent arrival had fueled it to a fever pitch. Apparently, no one wanted to be in the same room with the Evil Doctor who had the power to snuff out a life by merely pointing a bony finger at his selected victim and announcing his fate.

The staff's attempts at reasoning, cajoling, bribing, and even threatening their wards had failed. Walking down the corridors, my steps seemed to resonate from the tiled floors like Teutonic jackboots. My face at a patient's door evoked moaning from males and sobbing from females, both pulling bedclothes over their heads. I had run the gamut from room A-1 to B-15, confounded by this, when I glanced at my watch. *My God, it was 9:15!* I was a dead man because I had missed my surgical assignment.

All those hours of faithful service in the O.R., flashing my surgical skill to the pleasure of my mentors, my incredible diagnostic acumen at Grand Rounds, the covert hints at partnership from some of the Hospital Staff, all shot to hell. Who could respect someone who couldn't show up on time for scheduled surgery? A bald-faced lie about my wife's water breaking stuck in my throat, but finally slipped out.

You see, Your Honor, I had no choice but to offer this shameful prevarication, both to cover my own keister and to preserve the job for those who would follow.

Why the Chief of Service bought it, I'll never know, perhaps I was given a reprieve in light of my stellar past performance. That night, my first mirrored look at a certified liar repulsed me.

God's punishment was swift; my course was clear. The irreversible perception of me as a malevolent Motor City Mengèlc made the nursing home job untenable. Hence, my negotiation with a first-year resident; I expounded on the wisdom of accepting the nursing home gig in exchange for his job. He agreed, and I was soon driving into the nether parts of Crime City, U.S.A., to do those crappy insurance exams again.

I offhandedly suggested to my subordinate that, unless otherwise occupied, it would be prudent to keep his hands in his pockets. ✚

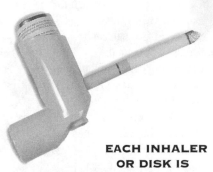
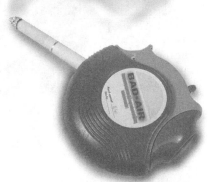

I was a resident in a Family Practice program in the early '80s. One of my assigned patients, whom we shall call Ann, was the type that would make me want to weep whenever I saw her name upon my schedule. Mercifully, her visits weren't frequent enough for me to require prescription antidepressants, so I just bit the bullet and got through each episode as best I could.

Ann never really had much of anything demonstrably wrong, but that never stopped diligent physicians from searching for the cause of her complaints. She had had multiple abdominal surgical procedures yet the surgical records either mysteriously vanished from her medical record or, when they hadn't disappeared, they reflected nebulous indications for the given procedure and questionable pathological findings from the procedure. Ann had convinced a neurologist that she had seizures and migraine headaches. Although narcotic requests were not part of her repertoire, Midrin (et al.) never seemed to quite do the job. And despite the fact that her seizure diagnosis was made totally by history, nobody had ever witnessed her having one. Her antiepileptic medication level never stayed in the therapeutic range unless she was an inpatient.

She got the E.R. physicians to admit her once for "seizures"; her low blood level of anticonvulsant medication seemed to bolster the need for this admission. By the time I saw her on the ward, she had convinced all of the staff that she needed extra padding on all the bed rails, headboards, etc. It was a sight to see, especially in view of the fact that she was always asleep when I came by . . . or should I say she appeared to be asleep. She would certainly be somnolent if there was any hint that a discussion about discharge from the hospital was about to take place.

THOSE DARN NARC SEEKERS

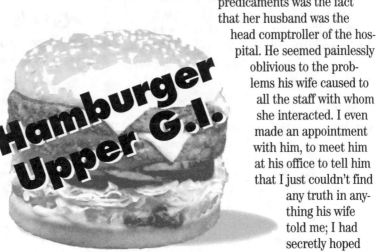

Hamburger Upper G.I.

Ironically, Ann became a volunteer in the hospital. This seemed commendable and innocent enough at first. However, she would go from doctor to doctor telling each one that one of the others had prescribed a diuretic for her and she needed a refill and would they be *so kind to write her one?* She was let go after two days on the job. There was no medical reason for her to need a diuretic; what made her seek them remains a mystery. I remain thankful that it wasn't a controlled drug she was seeking.

Complicating Ann's predicaments was the fact that her husband was the head comptroller of the hospital. He seemed painlessly oblivious to the problems his wife caused to all the staff with whom she interacted. I even made an appointment with him, to meet him at his office to tell him that I just couldn't find any truth in anything his wife told me; I had secretly hoped this would annoy them enough that they would seek a different doctor, but it didn't work.

One late November day Ann presented to my office reporting that she had been vomiting everything she had eaten for the previous two weeks. *Never mind that her physical exam showed nothing to support this. Never mind that her weight was unchanged. Never mind that some basic labs failed to support her contention.* Then it struck me. *"Ann, I saw you and your husband in the cafeteria on Thanksgiving Day and you appeared to be eating just fine."* She proceeded to tell me that that was the only meal in the last two weeks she hadn't vomited. *Imagine that!*

In an effort to look like I was doing something to investigate this vomiting, I told her I would get a test that would assess the anatomy and functionality of the stomach and upper intestinal tract. What I had in mind was a test we called a "**Hamburger Upper G.I.**" (*Does anybody still do this test?*) Call it Freudian if you wish, but after I had completed the request form, I discovered I had written an order for a "Hamburger Barium Enema"! I was half tempted to leave the order as (mis)written, just for punitive purposes!

Ann actually went through with the Hamburger Upper G.I. When she returned to my office to discuss the results, she went to great pains to describe to me how horrible the ordeal was and how she would have never made it through the test if one of my co-residents hadn't been there to hold her hand and encourage her the whole time. Of course, when I asked "Bill" for his version of what went on, it was nothing like her description; Bill essentially was passing through radiology and greeted Ann then went on his way. *The result of the test?* Normal, naturally.

After I left the residency, I had my first non-residency job as a Family Physician in a clinic about a mile from the hospital where I'd trained. *Gadzooks!* Ann showed up not long after that, much like the proverbial bad penny. Fortunately for me, she was not eligible for care at the clinic for administrative reasons. That didn't stop her from asking for a "curbside consult," but I felt comfortable deflecting it by requesting that she see her own doctor for such requests.

I only saw Ann once after that. She was working in a local department store; I only saw her there once and I took the coward's way out: I was able to pretend that I hadn't seen her lest she try to converse with me.

We've all had our dishonest and unreliable patients but for me, this one "takes the cake" . . . or should I say hamburger. ✚

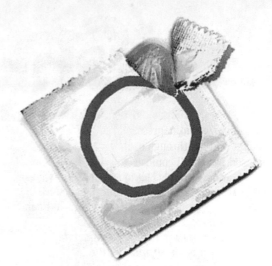

A LITTLE PREMATURE

I was a first-year resident doing free school physicals for poor farm kids in rural eastern Colorado. My fellow residents and I were taught to ask all the usual adolescent questions (drug use, alcohol use, sexual activity, etc.) when a large, healthy 17-year-old senior football player entered the room. I started my line of questioning for the 20th time that day when I got to my pat question, *"Are you sexually active?"* He replied with a hearty, *"Yea, of course I'm sexually active!"* My pat follow-up was, *"Are you using some form of protection . . . like condoms?"*

He replied, now rather sheepishly, ***"Well, I'm sexually active, but I haven't got that far yet."*** ✚

Shrunken Head

I was pretty goofy at the end of a 24-hour shift in the medical ER as an intern at a city hospital in 1966. The triage nurse informed me Mr. Block, a 47-year-old unmarried man, was in Room 12-B with the presenting complaint:

> *"Every time I smoke a cigarette, my penis shrinks a little bit!"*

I was tired and told the nurse to tell him to blow the smoke out his ass, and then his penis would get bigger every time instead of smaller. The old biddy did NOT think this was funny, and insisted he had to be seen before I left.

Mr. Block had his "poor shrunken" penis on display when I entered the room, made it clear he would not object to very thorough examination, and said he hoped I would be – finally – the doctor who could bring him a prospect of recovery!

THEN A CREATIVE THOUGHT STRUCK ME!

I explained to the patient baseline and post-cigarette consumption measurements would be essential before examination and said I would be back after these tests were completed.

Two cute little pure and innocent 18-year-old student nurses were always hovering by the nursing station ready to follow doctor's orders literally (*Those were the good old days!*), so in my most officious "high and mighty" doctor lingo I handed them Mr. Block's chart and said, ***"We have a possible case of Oro-Peno-Recto-Nicotine Stenosis in 12-B. This is quite rare!*** *Baseline measurements must include circumference and length of his penis (while pulled out as far as possible), then after you give him an enema take his rectal temperature leaving the thermometer in a full 5 minutes. Then allow him to smoke a cigarette of his choice, and 5 minutes after he is done measure circumference and length of his penis again, and then check rectal temperature again. [In that era, temperature was always taken rectally, for you young docs!] Bring me the measurements when you are done and we will decide what to do."*

 With ashen, horror-stricken faces, off the student nurses went to do their duty, and of course I retreated into the interns' and residents' lounge to entertain my (equally goofy) colleagues with this great story. I was also putting through a call to the local psychiatric hospital to send over some techs to haul the guy off into the nuthouse. *(We could actually do that way back then!)*

THEN THE BAD NEWS STRUCK!

The psych hospital intake nurse said: *"Oh, no, not Mr. Block again, no way! He does this act all over the state! He isn't ever coming back here again!"* I was starting to realize my "joke" was not so smart when the shrieking bellow of the ER Head Nurse could be heard halfway to Canada!

"Dr. Baarrr!"

Oh, she was hopping mad! The student nurses had been caught in the act of carrying out my orders when Mr. Block started screaming bloody murder. He didn't want any girls in his room pulling on his penis and giving him an enema! The Head Nurse found him curled up in a corner with a blanket pulled up to protect him against the students. She told me (and the other now very quiet interns and residents in the lounge) this was the same man who showed up in ERs all over the western part of the state every summer for the past 20 years with the same complaint. He knew there would always be a new shift of young doctors to try to entice into examining him, but she had never seen or heard of any intern or resident stupid or crazy enough to give whacko orders like I did!

The Chief of Medicine kind of hammered home that point the next day in his office, but then he paused for a moment and said, *"You know, this man has now been physically examined by hundreds of young male doctors over some 20 years, and there might be a lesson here for him. You ordered something he was totally unprepared for and did not expect. This might completely disrupt his long-standing pattern of malingering! I see here, in your record, you are applying to Yale, Harvard, University of Colorado, and Stanford for a psychiatric residency. Did you use a psychiatric perspective in ordering these crazy tests to disrupt his malingering pattern?"*

I gave great thought to my answer, but then answered honestly: *"No, sir. I was goofy, I was tired, there was a Code Blue in the ER that shift we pulled through and one I helped with upstairs in ICU we lost, and we had a 7-year-old brought into Peds ER in full arrest, everybody tried to help. The kid died an hour before this whacko showed up, and I got to be the one to tell his mother there was nothing more we could do, because I was the only intern applying for a psych residency. I had no patience left for a nut case like this. All I had left was a really wicked sense of humor."*

The chief thought this answer over, and said: *"Two senior residents there were evidently laughing right along with you, so I gather you had full collegial support. It was not a wise or conventional idea, but I can't and won't blame you for using it. Good day."*

So I posted a note in the ER doctors' lounge:
"By order of the Chief of Medicine, henceforth, all prospective cases of Oro-Peno-Recto-Nicotine Stenosis must first be evaluated at St. Mary's Catholic Hospital ER" (knowing all exams there would be done by nuns). *THOSE WERE THE "GOOD OLD DAYS!"*

UPDATE: When I was just a tired kid intern, I had no idea of the horror of the Pandora's Box I was opening when I played that little *"innocent"* joke. By the end of that academic year, all manner of sh*t had hit the fan. In fact, in my interviews for residency positions at Stanford, Yale, U. Colorado, Harvard, Cincinnati, and U. North Carolina, there were nasty questions about this incident – and my judgment, and my "problematic" impulsivity.

Tragically, a far more complete picture emerged over the next few months, and the case was presented and discussed at length at a combined Medicine/Psychiatry Grand Rounds in the fall of that year. It turned out the man was once a first-class ER nurse trained at a major university who lost his license four years prior, and had been hospitalized at as many as eight to ten psychiatric hospitals all over the

NE for similar complaints. He had evidently been seen for an assortment of pelvic complaints at many dozens of medical ERs all over, with visits mostly in the months of July, August, and September.

He used all manner of chief complaints, some very conventional such as suggesting inguinal hernia symptoms or VD; he apparently inflicted bruises and lacerations on his penis and testicles to require minor surgical attention; and then there were the more bizarre complaints such as he manifested when I saw him. I remember one reportedly was,

"I accidently slipped a glass drink stirring straw down my penis, and now I can't get it out!"

Further data emerged that he was amazingly careful and purposeful, to the point that he collected the names and pictures of all new medicine and surgery interns and residents, and found ways to ("innocently") connect with house staff scheduling personnel at dozens of hospitals in the area. Among the perhaps 250 house staff at the Grand Rounds, dozens of us were interns and residents who had seen him, and we were invited to stand. *It was instantly chilling!* The professor pointed out how we were all very "boyish," athletically built, seemingly "handsome" young men. **We had been purposely pre-selected.** He also wanted very naive and inexperienced interns and residents examining him, presuming this would lead to more thorough evaluations, and this was evidently why he usually went to ERs immediately after a new batch of interns and residents started training every summer.

Several wags at the Grand Rounds suggested an individual with a compulsion this severe could not possibly go as long as eight months every year between such gratifying examinations. The presenting professors agreed this was odd, indeed. In the late spring of the next year, an addendum was reported: the man was a dual American-Canadian citizen, and under a different name he evidently was on 10 to 15 evaluation lists for Medical School Urology clinics all over Ontario and Quebec, where he would be examined by young medical students! ✚

Problem?

One busy day before Thanksgiving, when I was an intern in Family Medicine at a large inner city hospital, a dressed-too-nice-to-be-in-my-clinic couple came in to talk with the physician on duty. She was a bank branch manager and he was the general manager of a local Toyota dealership. Our clinic nurse took the couple into the exam room, but she was unable to elicit any information from the couple about their complaint. She was not able to obtain any medical history, for that matter. My medical student and I entered the exam room and introduced ourselves; we encountered the patient, a well-kept middle-aged woman, sitting on the exam table. She appeared very anxious and nervous, wringing her hands; her patient husband was standing at her side.

I noticed that she had a brown paper department store bag at her feet.

Trying to impress my medical student with my ability to obtain information from paranoid patients, I asked some brief questions. I finally determined that the best reason for this patient's visit was that she was seeking medical help for a problem she had discovered. This being the afternoon before a major holiday, this was the only clinic that would see her on short notice. **Her vague complaint was that she had discovered that the FBI and the CIA, along with the local police department, and even hospital security, had a plan to take over the United States.**

Biting my bottom lip to keep from smiling where the patient could see, and looking smugly at my medical student, I asked the patient to detail this plot she had discovered.

After some assurance from me that she could trust me, she confided that the FBI and CIA were inoculating all family dogs with rabies in order to deteriorate our nation's healthcare system. **This action would devastate the United States population and enable them to take over the country.**

As I was doing my best not to start laughing at this point, the patient reached down to pick up her shopping bag and said,

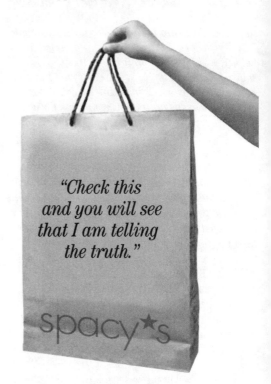

"Check this and you will see that I am telling the truth."

When I looked into the bag, it contained the head of her pet dog.

She requested that I check the dog's brains, and I would see the rabies.

I decided at this point that I would notify hospital security and arrange for an emergency commitment for the patient. Leaving the medical student alone in the exam room with the patient and her dog's head, I asked her husband to step into the hall with me to advise him of our plans for admission. After walking a few steps down the hall, away from the patient's ability to overhear, I looked at the patient's husband and asked bluntly, *"How long has your wife had this problem?"*

Without hesitation, he answered,

"What problem?" ✚

SLEEP STUDY

I was on call during Internal Medicine residency when the code pager alarmed at its usual hour, 4 a.m. I arrived to find the code underway on an elderly nursing home patient with multiple medical problems. Efforts were unsuccessful. Unfortunately, previous attempts to persuade the daughter to allow the ill patient to pass away naturally, without resuscitative efforts, had been equally unsuccessful.

The resident in charge of the patient was busy, so I told him I would contact the daughter and private attending. I hadn't worked with this attending extensively so I wasn't sure if he would want the "quick version" or all of the details. When he returned his page I gave him a synopsis of the patient's clinical deterioration that night and a recap of the code, ending with, "*. . . which was unsuccessful.*"

There was silence on the phone for long moments, then unexpectedly he sleepily asked, "*She's still intubated?*"

Stunned and admittedly confused, I stammered, "*Y-yes? . . .* "

"Get a pulm and cardio consult," was the reply.

Cutting through the confusion, I exclaimed,
**"*Doctor, I'm trying to tell you
the patient is DEAD!*"**

"*Oh . . . Okay.*" Click. Dial Tone.

I hung up the phone and walked over to some fellow residents who had been at the code. I must have had an uncharacteristically astonished look on my face, since they instantly stopped me to ask what the attending had said. In my usual deadpan I told them, "*He wants a pulmonary and cardiology consult.*"

Now they looked as disbelieving as I had been. I said, "*Either he was half-asleep or 'Covering Your Ass' has really gotten out of control.*" ✚

TEACHABLE MOMENT

M y story begins with the first case of the day in my residency procedure clinic. Ms. Chatterly, a 17-year-old female, has been referred to me for a colposcopy for cervical cancer. (The colposcope is a machine that allows us to look at a woman's cervix close up.) Her mom stayed long enough to sign the consent form and vanished. The young girl was not a patient I had seen before. I began by taking her history. Shortly after the history taking began she proceeded to start balling about, "*Why is this happening to me?*" We found out that her mother had had a hysterectomy at 25 years of age for cervical cancer. I was not surprised to discover that Ms. Chatterly had dropped out of school last year. As near as I could tell she had to quit school to pursue her other interests, which include smoking one to two packs of cigarettes per day and

spending time with her suitors. She had managed to encounter 12 to 15 sexual partners since age 13. I then recognized a "teachable moment" and had a LONG dialogue with her regarding her lifestyle choices as they related to her current condition.

The actual colposcopy with biopsies went about as expected. Strike that. There was more crying than I expected. Following the procedure I left to allow her to dress and to prepare my speech. When I returned I found her standing dressed and ready with coat on, her Marlboro Lights in one hand and lighter in the other. Before I even had a chance to speak, she asked, "*So Doc, how long do I have to wait before I have sex?*" I then forgot my speech, and calmly replied, "Three to four months." I didn't think she would believe a year. ✚

Whilst working in a busy trauma and burns ICU as a tired and permanently stressed resident, keeping my head above water was a Herculean task. The day-to-day grind of the job could be worsened by the arrival of my boss, a particularly toxic little surgeon who more than compensated for his small stature and male pattern baldness by being generally unpleasant to any unfortunate member of staff he came across. As is often the way with such people, he was unbelievably vain and wore the most fantastic (and expensive) hairpiece that money could buy.

The fact that the whole world could tell it was a wig

appeared not to have crossed his mind and he was often seen running his short, stubby fingers through his rug whilst gazing intermittently into any darkened window he passed. I will of course refer to him from now on as Dr. X.

On one particularly unpleasant day, a patient we had been ventilating and inotroping for a week following a nasty house fire started to decompensate. Oxygenation became difficult and the chest X-ray showed the severe ARDS (acute respiratory distress syndrome) we had been expecting for days. All ventilatory maneuvers failed to resolve the problem and I called Dr. X to avail him of the situation. He reviewed the case notes and radiology and announced to us that he wanted the patient turned to the prone position.

Turning a ventilated patient prone involves a significant coordination of manpower to ensure that all those carefully placed lines and tubes are not pulled out or dislodged. To his credit, Dr. X rolled up his sleeves and donning a gown offered to help with the head end during the turn.

Myself and a group of nurses prepared the lines and on Dr. X's word disconnected the ventilator and began to turn the patient.

Unfortunately for my esteemed boss, I had failed to put the ventilator into its standby mode after disconnecting and the machine (only following it's programming, I suppose) sensed a drop in airway pressure and tried to compensate by delivering an almighty breath from the disconnected tubing.

To my horror, a huge spray of pulmonary secretions (which had been hiding in the tubing and filter) shot into my boss's face and lifted the front inch of his toupee from his forehead!

the wig

The silence that followed seemed to last forever as we desperately tried to complete both our proning maneuver and turn off the flailing ventilator. At least two more blasts of secretion covered Dr. X who, as he was holding the airway, was unable to move out of the way.

After we had finished (and I had tried to apologize at least twenty times), my boss, a bright shade of crimson, walked off the ward and toward the changing rooms. As he went through the door into the corridor every nurse and respiratory tech in the unit started to laugh. He slowed his pace as if to turn, but then hurried out.

I had another month of burns to suffer prior to moving to another position and in all my remaining weeks my relationship with Dr. X remained curt but polite.

The incident was never mentioned, although the wig changed. ✚

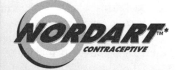

MY FAVORITE
MUNCHAUSEN

Pheobe was in the nursing field. She had a bad case of hypertension. It seemed that whatever medication the doctors would try would eventually fail. Soon Pheobe began having hypertensive crises. The headaches, tachycardia and sweating were unbearable for her. This is where our story starts.

A little background on Pheobe first, however. She had three miscarriages in the past due to increased blood pressure and high blood sugar. Her only delivery of a normal child had the complication of severe eclampsia (hypertension in pregnancy/delivery). She stated that her father died in his 50s due to a hypertensive crises as did five of her siblings from the same problem in their 50s as well. *Hmm.* Obviously, a genetic component was at work here.

Prior to our authors getting a hold of Pheobe, investigations were performed at many different hospitals. Catecholamine testing, 24-hour urine testing, clonidine inhibition tests, MIBG scintigraphy, CT of the abdomen, and MRI of the abdomen were all done to find the cause of Pheobe's duress. *No luck.* Much of the same tests were performed not once more, but twice more, and again no answer. Finally, Pheobe made her way to our hero's den.

She didn't look well. She was about 130 pounds. Actually, that was about it. Everything else on exam was completely normal. Her blood pressure of 140/80 mmHg was pretty good as well. Then the blood testing began. Everything was normal except the adrenaline and noradrenaline were way out of whack. This lady had a pheochromocytoma! *Forget horses, we have a zebra here.*

Our authors now began their diagnostic studies. Ultrasound of the throat and abdomen were normal. CT of the neck, thorax, abdomen and pelvis were normal. MRI of the abdomen was normal. MIBG scintigraphy and arteriography was also normal.

Soon our friends began taking venous blood samples to find the location of this pheochromocytoma. This tumor which causes extreme hypertension needed to be found immediately. Luckily an "enhance-

ment" showed up in the right adrenal gland and soon it was removed surgically. *Wouldn't you know it but under the microscope the adrenal gland was normal?* Even worse, Pheobe's hypertension crises were continuing.

By this point Phoebe was getting pissed. Up to six hypertensive crises were occurring a day. Her doctors were running tests and doing useless surgeries and they were finding nothing. She must have thought them incompetent. They tried every blood pressure medicine they could find, even ones not available in her country, and yet there was still failure.

The doctors tried testing all over again and were stumped once more. Then something showed up. A glimmer of hope. The concentration of adrenaline and noradrenaline were exceptionally high in left adrenal vein. Due to more life-threatening blood pressure crises, the surgeons were called and the decision was made to take out Pheobe's left (and last) adrenal gland. It was go time.

Like a miracle, something showed up out of nowhere and in the nick of time to stop the surgery. A clue had unearthed itself to spare Pheobe another useless procedure. *Thank goodness.* It seems the medical staff had found bottles of noradrenaline and adrenaline as well as syringes (some half-filled) around Pheobe's bedside. *Hurray!*

So here is how she did it. Pheobe would take the syringe and with perfect timing inject herself intravaginally. *Ouch!* She would even pull this trick off during some of the diagnostic studies! When she was confronted, Pheobe denied all. In fact, her hypertensive crises got worse and more frequent right after the confrontation. A forced admission to a psychiatric ward under constant surveillance cured everything. *Who says "Big Brother" is always a bad thing?* No more hypertensive crises were ever found.

Pheobe couldn't stay forever. Eventually she was discharged and off to visit another hospital of her choice. Our authors ended their discussion by stating that they had heard Phoebe "had developed a new Munchausen syndrome." Good luck Pheobe and let's hope you can be a little more careful next time. ✚

Liberally adapted and embellished from the European Journal of Medical Research *(1998) 3:549-553.*

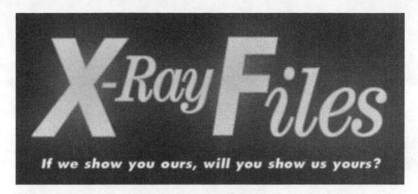

THROCKMORTEN SIGN WITH A TWIST

Riddle: A 26-year-old man was X-rayed for hip pain. There was no pathology found. MRI was not advised!

Answer: Metal things are pulled really hard in the MRI scanner. OUCH!

A gay friend of mine tells me it's called a *Prince Albert* – derivation unknown.

EDITOR'S <u>NOTE</u>: Does it have anything to do with getting Prince Albert in the can?

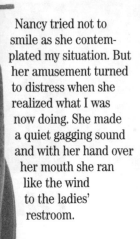

During my residency I found myself with some time on my hands one long call night. (*I know what you are thinking, this cannot be a true story because what resident has time on their hands?*) But indeed it is true and I swear to you that it did occur. You can ask my victims.

I was eating peanut butter when it occurred to me that the texture, color, and viscosity resembled something I had encountered on a proctology rotation. With this inspired thought, I carefully applied about two tablespoons of chunky style to the side and sole of my right shoe. I added a small smear of strawberry jam and I was off to the Emergency Department in search of a victim who would provide me with the reaction I craved.

I spotted Nancy, a registered nurse of long experience and a finely tuned and accurate bullshit meter. She smiled at me pleasantly and then turned as I addressed her.

"Oh man, look at that will you? I can't believe I got that on me!"

I yelled while pointing and looking down at my shoe.

"What is that?" Nancy asked, her eyes wide with horror at my anticipated reply.

"What does it look like? It's shit!

I shouldn't have walked into that guy's room; diarrhea all over the floor, the bed, the walls . . . aarrhhhggghh!!!"

Nancy tried not to smile as she contemplated my situation. But her amusement turned to distress when she realized what I was now doing. She made a quiet gagging sound and with her hand over her mouth she ran like the wind to the ladies' restroom.

Mission accomplished, I retreated to my call room after **I finished licking the rest of the peanut butter and jam off my shoe via my right index finger.**

I heard later that Nancy did not emerge from the restroom for the better part of thirty minutes, pale and diaphoretic, with a few choice observations about my character, my intelligence, and lack of class.

The remaining nurses on the shift made my life a living hell for the rest of the night and well into the next day as they called me for orders which were not necessary, which they normally handled, and strategically spaced in time so as to interrupt the maximum amount of REM sleep possible. I didn't mind though, what's another lost night of sleep compared to the sheer joy of completely disgusting an ER nurse?

It doesn't get much better than that. ✚

NEVER TOO LATE

As a resident with three months to go in residency, patience with patients begins to run on the short side. Taking call becomes a little less educational and a bit more . . . well, let's say laborious. Although I'm not complaining about resident's pay . . . but a night of moonlighting is a stark difference.

At 8 p.m. on the evening of a Sunday night call, I received a call from the nurse requesting me to speak with a 35-year-old female with the complaint of diarrhea for eleven days. Covering for some twenty staff physicians, I had no idea who this person was, but by this time in residency I had come to know the type of patients that her staff doctor seemed to attract. A quick scan on the computer showed that this patient suffered from irritable bowel syndrome (IBS) and depression to name a few problems.

Over the phone, the patient relayed that she was having a flare of her IBS resulting in four to five "blowout" stools a day. The patient had been ordered by the staff's nurse to try Lomotil to control the diarrhea but to call the office or go to the ER if the Lomotil did not work. So, here we are 11 days into this "flare" and she is calling me to get permission to go the ER . . . I mean she had taken a whole three Lomotil today and had "failed" her therapy!!!

In what amounted to be a twenty-five minute phone conversation to map out a plan of attack for this patient, I tried to point out that waiting another twelve hours for the clinic to open would be wiser than "utilizing" the ER. My main point was that it would be at least $500 cheaper to wait.

"Oh no," she exclaimed, *"it won't cost me a penny because I have Medicaid."*

I blurted out,

"Medicaid is not free, I pay for it!"

Oops, not the best thing to say to an unstable, depressed patient with "explosive" diarrhea.

Amazingly the comment slid by . . . or so I thought. Twenty minutes later the nurse calls again stating that the patient wishes to speak to me directly. She had reviewed her notes of our conversation and now had become offended. She requested an apology, which I was quick to give . . . but I also made sure she understood Medicaid is not a free ticket (at least for those who have to pay).

Now I wait . . . wait for the next phone call – that being the one from my program director.

Even with three months left, it really isn't too late to learn! ✚

THE NEW DOCTOR

INTRODUCTION

Hooray! The new doctor is here! The new doctor is here!

Unfortunately, this is something only heard on corny television shows and in movies. In reality, there are no grand celebrations and there are no red carpets. Sure, some hospitals may have a lame welcome party for the new blood coming in each year, but that is basically all you get. The doctors on staff may smile and say hello the first day, but the next day you are on your own. *"Good to have you with us"* is what they say, but ***"Get your ass to work"*** is what they mean. This is usually capped off by putting you on-call your first weekend on the job. On-call is the despised responsibility of being at the whim and mercy of patients as well as the emergency department. In fact, my first night on call was a classic example of what's in store for new physicians.

It was my first week in practice and I was raw as could be. I was called to the ER because a patient, who had no primary care doctor, had a fever. This was no big deal except for the fact that he had had a kidney transplant in the past. Not knowing how to "turf him" to a specialist yet, I went in and did the job. To turf someone means to pass off the patient to another physician more capable than you are or who should be doing the job instead of you. **I didn't know any better, so I worked my ass off for hours.** I tried to remember everything I'd ever been taught about long-term transplant effects and problems. I called the transplant center at the teaching hospital in the next state and got their advice. They were nice enough to go over everything – what I knew and what I'd never known – with me. After finishing up and tying the loose ends into a nice package, I decided to call our local nephrologist (kidney doctor) and alert her of the admission. I figured she could stay in bed and come in and consult in the morning. I was still, at that time in my life, very considerate.

"Did you take care of renal transplant patients where you trained!" she yelled.

"No."

"Then what makes you think you can take care of them now!"

"I don't know. I did call the transplant center and they . . . "

"I'm coming in," she interrupted and hung up on me.

The ER doctor turned pale when I told him that the nephrologist was on her way. *"Oh, boy,"* he muttered as he walked away scratching his head. ***Now I knew why he called me in the first place to admit the patient!*** I convinced myself that I wasn't scared of her, but did find myself sneaking out the back exit a short time later anyway. I didn't need to be berated again in person on my first call night.

All in all, though, it was an important lesson and I learned it well: **Some doctors are nice and some are pricks – the key to surviving medicine is determining who is who.** In fact, to this day, I still don't speak to this nephrologist, and I can confidently say it hasn't made my life any worse. She is still a witch and now I am mocking her in print. It's sweet justice for me.

Every doctor goes through similar rites of passage on the road to becoming a real physician. Each doctor's experience is unique, and obviously, it is not all bad. For most doctors it is an exciting new step in life; a huge threshold to cross. Leaving residency for a new position in a new location is a breath of fresh air. More importantly, you finally feel that you are somebody; that you made it in life. You look forward to proving your worth. You know you are smart and well-trained and you want to show it to all the other doctors in town. You want to make a difference in the world and be part of that medical "club." But you are still the new kid on the block, and don't know yet what you don't know, as my first on-call experience showed.

As a new doctor, you have a unique set of insecurities. You wonder to yourself whether you really are good enough. You are unsure of your decisions. Do you know enough to be independent? You ask yourself, *"Oh my God, no one is going to check on me?"* When you talk to other doctors, you are nervous because you question whether they are scrutinizing you or not. **The truth is they are.** It takes time to feel comfortable with the new kid on the block. You are a rookie to them and the only way to build their trust is to work with them over many years. The same thing is true with the nurses you meet. Until you prove your worth to them they will deem you incompetent. If they like you they will try to "train" you to be the doctor they want to work with: pleasant, responsive, and open to their suggestions. **If they don't like you they conspire with other nurses to make your life a living hell.**

Even patients get in on this training process. Initially, every new doctor gets to see lots and lots of new patients. New doctors are always very popular. Unfortunately, lots and lots of these patients are doctor shoppers looking for a new miracle worker or a narcotic supplier. Like flies attracted to fresh stool, these patients block up your schedule for months until you get wise to the whole game and send them back to wherever they came. It's all part of the initiation.

With time, things do get a lot better. Call is easier as compared to the hell you went through in residency. You have on average over $100,000 in student loans so you can use the income. You even have extra money to spend on yourself and even on your family . . . *and spend you will!* The patients seem a lot nicer. In fact, you start to question why Old Dr. Hibbard was so bitter when he retired and left you his practice. With time you get more comfortable in your new role as real doctor. Until then, however, you are a blank canvas waiting to be filled up with open abscesses, pelvic exams gone wrong, vomit in your face, legs that fall off, and kids that punch you in your crotch. It is these experiences, as well as some of the others depicted in the following stories, which become the foundation of your medical career.

No one ever said it was going to be easy.

✚

Starting out in practice is not so easy. The learning curve is high and the confidence level is low because you are finally on your own. I was seeing a patient new to my practice one early autumn morning.

Mr. Raymond was a very nice older gentleman and seemed happy to see me. I am a female family practitioner and Mr. Raymond was not only very jovial, but a little flirtatious. This didn't bother me as he really was harmless – *or so I thought.*

He had a very complicated medical history and since he was transferring to me, I wanted to impress him with my skill. *Don't we all put on a little show when someone comes to us because their other physician let them down in some manner?* I really spent a tremendous amount of time obtaining a complete history which included everything from diabetes to heart disease with a little touch of COPD. I delved into the past treatment of each ailment and even impressed myself with my thoroughness. I thought to myself,

"I'm pretty good at this."

When it came to his exam I was determined to be perfect, but time was not on my side. I didn't have him fully undress because it wasn't set up as a complete physical. As I was trained, I started at the top and worked my way down to his toes. Nothing seemed to be that unusual until I got to his extremities.

As stated earlier, this man was a diabetic and I wanted to see if he had good circulation in his lower limbs. When I got to his pedal pulses, I found none in his left foot. I must admit, this part of the exam is not my strength, but I really couldn't feel anything. I quickly replayed his history to remind myself if he had told me about any peripheral vascular disease. He didn't. I think.

"Any problems with your left leg?" I asked.

"No, Doc. Why, is there a problem?" he replied.

This is where it got tricky. I had to admit that either he had a compromised leg or I just couldn't feel pedal pulses very well.

This was not the best way to build up confidence in your new patient. I shared my dilemma with him. At that point he kindly offered to remove his sock.

Chatting nonchalantly all along, the sock comes off with a little effort *and then so does his entire calf!* I let out a little girly scream and Mr. Raymond burst out laughing and proceeds to yell,

"I GOTCHA!"

The fact that he neglected to inform me of his left below-the-knee amputation was a slight oversight on both our parts. He stated that he makes a point of doing it to all the new young female doctors he meets and they fall for it every time. Needless to say, Mr. Raymond soon became my new favorite patient and I now always have my diabetics take their off socks during the exam. ✚

WINDY

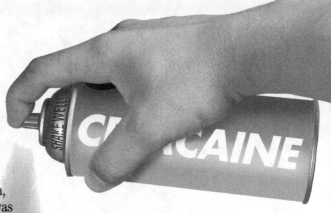

A 17-year-old girl comes in to the ER with pelvic pain, dysuria, and a discharge. She had been in two days prior and saw one of the other docs, but the medication he prescribed hadn't helped. She did not allow a pelvic exam the previous visit and would only allow a nurse to do a swab for a wet prep. She demanded that there be no speculum, no physician, and no gynecological. She was planning to get married in five days. Her mom was in the room with her and I told both of them that basically she had failed the presumptive treatment given by the other doctor. There needed to be a pelvic exam if she wanted any legitimate treatment for whatever is going on. The girl began to freak out.

"KNOCK ME OUT! YOU'VE GOT TO KNOCK ME OUT!"

"I'm not going to knock you out for a pelvic exam," I stated.

"WELL THEN, MAKE IT NUMB OR SOMETHING."

"No, there's nothing that's going to make it numb."

"THERE'S GOT TO BE SOMETHING, A CREAM OR SPRAY OR SOMETHING?!?"

"No, there's really not anything like that for this examination." She carried on like this for a while (in the stirrups of course, and Mom holding her hand compassionately).

"YOU'VE GOT TO DO SOMETHING. THERE HAS TO BE A SPRAY OR SOME SORT OF MEDICINE!"

In the meantime, I'm losing my patience, the ER is swamped, and I say *"Fine, there is a spray but it will burn so bad you'll wish it had never happened."*

"I DON'T CARE. USE THE SPRAY. MAKE IT NUMB!"

So I get a can of cetacaine and give her two good sprays.

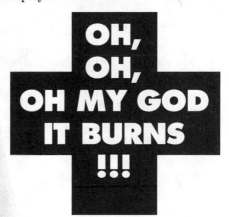

OH, OH, OH MY GOD IT BURNS !!!

"BLOW ON IT!! BLOW ON IT!"

I'm not kidding, word for word.
No, I did not blow on it.
I guess cetacaine isn't such a wonderful drug on open herpetic lesions.

So everyone in the ER busts a gut over this and mocks me nearly every time I come to work. I even had a neurosurgeon make a crack the other day. *"How's it going Puff Daddy?"* ✚

TOP TEN

Clues That You Are NOT Getting Your Patient, John Squatter, Out of the Hospital Today

10 The satellite guy for Direct TV is hooking up a unit outside John's window.

9 You receive an invitation for a 4th of July party (3 months away) with directions to the hospital and, more specifically, John's room.

8 You try to enter the room but it is locked and a new doorbell has been installed.

7 You see a sign above the door, "Welcome to John's Place."

6 John's family has begun to move in their own furniture.

5 Like a squirrel, John has begun hoarding food and other stuff into piles around the room.

4 Preprinted envelope stickers for John Squatter have arrived from the *Disabled Veterans of Any War* charity.

3 Color samples of drapery and linens are left around the room by the interior decorator John has recently hired.

2 AMWAY has begun meeting in the room and John has reached "Triple Diamond" by selling to the nurses.

1 Telemarketers keep interrupting your exam to ask if John Squatter would be interested in changing long distance plans.

JUST CAN'T GET PREGNANT

While working in a small community in Kansas, an established patient came in for an office visit for lower abdominal pain. She was a married, 31-year-old white female who was obese and not very sharp. She also had buck teeth that were an unusual shade of yellow. During the history and physical, I asked if there was a possibility she could be pregnant to rule out this being a possible cause of her abdominal pain. She replied "*No.*"

"*Oh,*" I said, "*then you're on the pill?*"

"*No,*" she said.

"*Oh,*" I said "*then you have had your tubes tied or your husband has been fixed?*"

"*No,*" she replied, "*I just can't get pregnant and my husband and I have been trying for the last five years.*"

Noticing she was upset with this, I told her that there was a chance that it might be her husband who is not able to produce children.

"*No,*" she said, "*all of his friends have tried and it didn't work either, so I know it is me.*" ✚

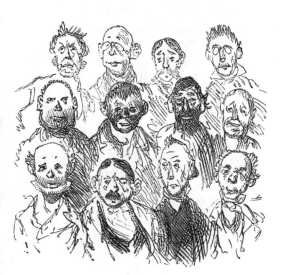

HERE'S ONE WAY TO BEAT THE SYSTEM

During my first year in private practice, I had a 20-year-old woman come to see me for a localized left breast infection. I initially put her on antibiotics and requested that she follow up with me in three days.

Three days later she came back in. The examination of her left breast showed not only was the infection spreading, but now there was a fluctuant mass there as well. I incised and drained the area and sent away for the appropriate cultures.

A few days later the results came back showing some type of bizarre anaerobic microbe that could not have possibly gotten there by any natural means. *Something smelled funny.* The next time I saw the patient I confronted her with the culture results. After a moment she broke down and started crying. She stated that she worked as a tech in the microbiology department of the local hospital. She desperately wanted some time off so she picked up a sample culture, scraped up some of the growth, put it in a TB syringe and injected into her left nipple area. The mystery was solved as we now had the reason for the impossible culture and a new method of getting worker's comp.

It was my first year in practice. She was new to the area. Her husband was in the military and they had just moved back to the states from the Orient. Her migraines were tortuous and she couldn't take it anymore. She needed something but nothing seemed to work.

She looked like she was going into labor her pain was so bad.

Joanne was a young and attractive woman. She was in her late twenties and already had a hysterectomy for chronic abdominal pain. *Hmm, that seemed weird.* I tried everything for her head. All the new migraine medications didn't touch them. The shots, nasal spray, and pills were like water to Joanne. Then it hit me. Maybe there was an estrogen component to her exacerbations. We tried adjusting her hormone therapy but wouldn't you know it, she kept coming in for narcotics. *That was the one constant medicine that would make her headaches go away.*

Something was always fishy to me about Joanne. Her symptoms were so overdramatic that each time was like an Oscar performance. Add to this that I could never get her records from the military doctors from overseas and my suspicions continued to grow.

I finally sent her to a neurologist who started the process all over again. MRIs, triptans, and even different types of birth control pills weren't the answer. Unfortunately, the neurologist never got to the bottom of the story either. Even though he started from scratch in the whole process, he ended up in the same dead end that I did.

Pretty soon Joanne started working both of us for her severe migraines and need for more and more narcotics. Whenever we hesitated she

THOSE DARN NARC SEEKERS

would either get very angry or make us feel guilty as hell for not finding an answer to her ordeal.

At some point, both the neurologist and I had had enough and we got a little tougher on Joanne. We said that she needed to get her medications from only one source. Unfortunately, the neurologist pointed her back my way as her source. *That sucked.* As I continued to try to regulate Joanne's use (or abuse?), she suddenly disappeared. *Trust me, I didn't try to find her.*

It was not until months later that my OB-GYN colleague was calling me and questioning about Joanne and her new abdominal pain. I had no idea why she would be going to an OB-GYN as she no longer had reproductive organs. Anyway, I passed along my stories of her migraines and her need for narcotics and we ended the conversation there.

Months later I was admitting a patient in the ED when I heard violent screaming. The EMTs were scurrying by the ambulance entrance. I saw them race the stretcher past me like the issue was life threatening. I caught a glimpse of the poor patient and it turned out to be Joanne. *Again, she looked like she was going into labor her pain was so bad.* None of the ED staff even moved. I saw the ED doc who was completely indifferent to the loud shrieks and she stated that Joanne had been making the rounds more frequently to get narcotics. Our little friend had now exhausted the last route of getting painkillers (that being the generous ED) since they were immune to her act. For me, it was surreal to see the EMTs running like chickens with their heads cut off and ED staff not even getting up. *Only a narc seeker has that ability to produce this type of reaction.*

I never saw Joanne again.

I don't believe she goes to our ED anymore or any other local doctor. She probably has moved, and unless she has detoxed, I recommend you think twice about giving narcotics to an overdramatic actress whose past is buried in the Orient.

✚

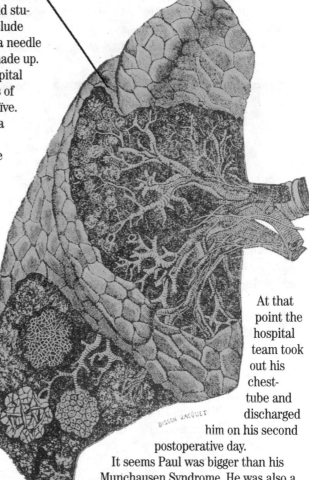

PAUL THE POPPER

Don't you ever find yourself popping those bubble wrapping papers? It can be quite addicting. I just love them. In some small way it relieves stress. This Munchausen has a similar addiction. He's a 30-year-old student that loves to travel. His hobbies include skiing, singing in the choir, and putting a needle in his chest. Actually, the first two are made up.

"Paul the Popper" came into the hospital complaining of chest pain and shortness of breath. *A heart attack you say?* How naïve. The X-rays show that his right lung had a pneumothorax or was punctured.

Paul had undergone many chest-tube insertions in his life for this problem because, as luck would have it, he kept getting spontaneous pneumo-thoraces. He had been seen in three different cities (at least) for this before. This time the physicians decided not to put in a chest-tube immediately as they felt the lung would reinflate on its own. Unfortunately, a recheck on the next X-ray showed that the lung was even smaller. The funny thing, however, was that something else was in the lung cavity as well. Wouldn't you know it, Paul had gotten a hypodermic needle stuck in his chest!

Talk about your bad days.

When they confronted Paul, he was incensed. *"This hospital should be ashamed of itself for leaving needles recklessly around the patient's bed!"*

This didn't stop our heroes from doing their job and taking Paul to the operating room to remove his needle, as well as part of his lung.

Heck, a 30-year-old doesn't need all that much lung tissue anyway.

"Paul the Popper," with enough prompting, finally admitted to his hobby of dropping a lung for fun. Yes, Paul was a Munchausen, but must all patients be given a label? They are so much more than one diagnosis. Our friend Paul was also caught stealing narcotics.

At that point the hospital team took out his chest-tube and discharged him on his second postoperative day.

It seems Paul was bigger than his Munchausen Syndrome. He was also a narc-seeker. Goodbye Paul, and we hope you find another city to float around in. *Don't forget your needles.* ✚

Ann Thorac Surg *2001;72:281-83.*

87

In the ongoing effort to save money, our 100 member medical group changed transcription services. It now goes through the Internet to India where it is transcribed and sent back within hours. No doubt we are contributing to a host of slave labor, but the cost was too good to pass up. Unfortunately, there is something lost in the translation as this next example will demonstrate.

One of my partners had wanted to dictate just how horrific his patient's car accident was and included the statement,

"The patient then had to be extricated with the jaws of life."

You and I, of course, can picture the frantic paramedics cutting through the rooftop to reach this surely critical patient.

When the dictation came back and was proofread (which now we really have to do!), the above line was interpreted as,

"The patient then had to be educated on the joys of life." ✚

About thirty years ago when I started my practice in psychiatry, I was on the staff of six different hospitals throughout the area. One was a small hospital that had the phone operator work as the admitting clerk during the night shift.

A young black lady with sickle cell anemia and depression was admitted, a consult was called, and I saw her the next day. I pulled her chart and flipped open to the admitting diagnosis of *"sick as hell anemia"*; a truer diagnosis was never made. ✚

We admitted a lady to the gynecology ward for vaginal bleeding. She filled out her paperwork and acknowledged that she was being admitted for
"Bleeding from my Virginia."

She was such a sweet (although under-educated) woman that I couldn't bring myself to correct her. ✚

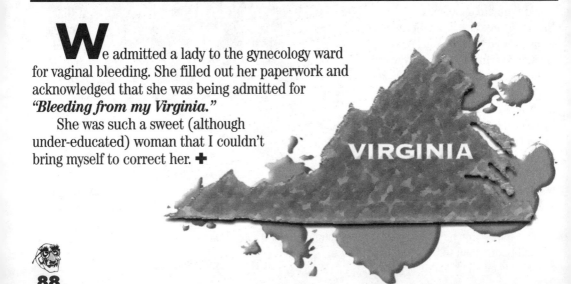

VIRGINIA

PROBLEMS

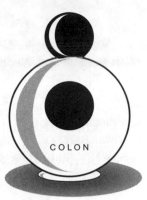

COLON

While taking a family history, a man told me that his sister had *"cancer of the cologne."* My immediate supposition was that it probably smelled better that way. ✚

A rather backwoods appearing woman informed me, as I was about to listen to her heart, that she had been told by previous doctors that she had a *"heart wormer."*

After confirming that what I thought I'd heard was indeed what she had said, I wondered if having her see a veterinarian might be more appropriate. ✚

VOICE RECOGNITION BLUES

I had recently obtained voice-recognition software for my computer and was dictating a note about a patient's visit. A lady had come to the office for a follow-up visit to evaluate how she was doing with her pessary. Pessaries are used in women who have a prolapsed vagina and need something to keep it from coming out all the time. They either use the pessary or get surgery. The software unfortunately misunderstood some of what I said:

"Patient comes in for a pussy check. Has no complaints. On exam, her pussy appears to be appropriately placed and functioning well. Her pussy is removed, cleaned and replaced without difficulty."

More recently, a different patient was interested in artificial insemination. Her note read:

"Patient presents requesting information regarding artificial insemination using donor seamen."

I recommend proofreading all your voice-recognition notes as some editing is definitely required. ✚

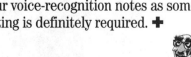

One evening on my ER shift, the head nurse came at me, chart in hand and devilish grin on her face. *"This one is a special for you, doctor!"* Assuming I was in for big trouble but not knowing exactly for what, I perused the chart. My eye fell on the chief complaint: *"Hot dog stuck in vagina."* The nurse asked if she should accompany me while I got the history, but I decided I'd do that portion alone.

On the table sat a middle-aged, bottle-blonde, chubby woman who appeared a bit restless. I introduced myself and proceeded to get some details.

*"Well, uh, you know, my husband has been away for about six months and, well, uh, you know, I needed some relief so I was 'doing' myself with this hot dog when I lost my grip and it went up inside. **And I can't get it out!** Oh, I can get my fingers on it but I keep losing my grip and now I've got myself sore from pulling on it!"*

I kept a professional demeanor and got the nurse for an exam. Standard speculum exam of the vagina was normal: normal vagina, normal cervix, no foreign object. Bimanual exam confirmed this but, as my gloved fingers moved her cervix, she said, *"There! You've got it – I can feel it!"*

HOT DIGGITY DOG!

I gave her cervix a gentle tug and asked her if this was what she was feeling when she was trying to pull out the "hot dog." *"Yes,"* she replied, *"can you remove it?"*

After explaining to her that what she was attempting to do was essentially a trans-vaginal hysterectomy, I reassured her that there was nothing within her lower reproductive tract that needed removal. She then asked in all sincerity, if the hot dog *"could have gone up further."*

We held a quick anatomy lesson, focusing on the diameter of the typical cervical canal versus the diameter of the typical hot dog. Naturally, she then asked me the question I couldn't answer: *"**Well, then where IS the hot dog?**"*

I could only speculate as to where the weenie could be, figuring that as long as it wasn't inside her, there wasn't anything further I could do. ✚

It was my first year of residency and I was on the OB-GYN service. To "gain more experience" we were sent to the ER for all problems related to this very special field of medical endeavor.

Late one Saturday night, the beeper went off and when I returned the call, the ER nurse reported that a young female complaining of vaginal bleeding was waiting for my evaluation. As I proceeded to the ER, my mind went through the multiple possible causes of vaginal bleeding, but I have to admit that I hadn't come up with what I was soon to be confronted with!

I entered the exam room with a nurse to find a "professional sex therapist" from the inner city neighborhood of our hospital.

She was somewhat reticent to describe her problem and so we helped her get into position for examination *(a position apparently not foreign to this young lady)*.

Upon insertion of the speculum and focusing the light on her introitus, I was presented with

a brown furry-appearing object and an intense odor

that drew an exclamation of surprise and revulsion from the nurse standing behind me.

Being the professional that I was, I turned and drew a deep breath and then armed with a ring forceps to prod the beast, went back in for another look.

As I grasped the brown fuzz within the vagina it began to break away and behind it deeper in the vault was more. Piece by piece I was able (with much breath holding) to extract the first of seven,

yes seven, tampons!

Intermingled within the brownish oozy mass, I also encountered a whitish suspiciously stretchy material. It was, yes, you guessed it,

the first of two condoms!

I never did discover any bleeding but there was considerable vaginitis evident after the foreign bodies were all removed. When I left the room to go write a prescription for the patient, Garbage Can Lady got dressed and was gone before I returned.

EDITOR'S NOTE:
We frequently get stories about retained tampons so they are not very interesting to publish. This one with seven, however, breaks the new world record and therefore we felt it needed to be published. Here's a toast to you, Garbage Can Lady! ✚

GARBAGE CAN LADY

Life on the Farm

It's not a joke.

I always thought these types of jokes were funny but never believed they were true. I mean, is it anatomically possible? Isn't it just folklore and legend? Well, more about this later.

Mr. Harold was 83 years old and extremely hard of hearing. I didn't know him as I was covering for my partner who was off for the day. The ER gave me the heads up that this gentleman had something wrong with him neurologically. He had woken up feeling "drunk" and had to lie back in bed quickly because of imbalance. His son and wife were very worried and called the ambulance later that morning to get him seen at the hospital.

. . . she knew why her husband was sick.

The ER doc said the patient was swaying to his right and kept losing his balance. His finger-to-nose testing was also off on the right. All other parts of the exam were normal including X-rays, labs, and CT of the head. By the time I saw the patient his symptoms were gone. This was late on a Friday and I admitted him overnight to have some ultrasound done on his carotids and an ECHO for a probable TIA (transient ischemic attack, or mini-stroke). *Of course, the best laid plans . . .*

He seemed like a nice guy. When he did hear, he answered the questions correctly and without any mental status changes.

My partner began seeing him on the following Monday and was told by the weekend cover that this man was ready to go. When he was examined and being packaged for discharge, he casually mentioned that when he got home he was going to blow his head off. *Where this came from no one knows.* He didn't look depressed to me when I saw him.

He was smiling and ready and excited to get out of the hospital. Maybe it was the hospital stay itself that was driving him to suicide or maybe he had other issues.

The patient was transferred to the psychiatric floor to be seen by the appropriate specialists. Prior to his being transferred, the nurse on the floor called my partner. She stated she just received the weirdest call. The patient's wife stated that she knew why her husband was sick. For twenty years he had been

"screwing all the animals on the farm. He screws the cow, the pigs and the sheep!"

This story is interesting on many levels. For one, why does the wife think his illness is due to having sex with the farm animals? Secondly, why does the wife let him have sex with farm animals? Does she still have sex with him knowing that he courts the sheep and longs for the pigs? Third, why does he want to blow his head off? Does he miss Claribelle, the cow with the pretty face? Maybe Claribelle is cheating on him with the bull or even worse, his neighbor Clem. Fourth, can he get an STD from having sex with these animals? Fifth, what the hell do we as physicians do with this couple?

My partner took this information into the patient's room the next day and was intending, out of morbid curiosity, to see what makes his farm animals so attractive. Rushed for time and probably struck with a brilliant flash of repulsion, he never addressed this issue. For the time being, Mr. Harold will continue to have his way with the "girls" in the barn and all we can do as physicians is to let the world know.

+

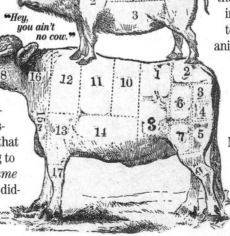

"Hey, you ain't no cow."

IN THE NAVY

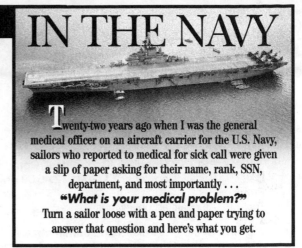

Twenty-two years ago when I was the general
medical officer on an aircraft carrier for the U.S. Navy,
sailors who reported to medical for sick call were given
a slip of paper asking for their name, rank, SSN,
department, and most importantly . . .
"What is your medical problem?"
Turn a sailor loose with a pen and paper trying to
answer that question and here's what you get.

A small penis, infection
(Two problems, I guess)

vitamin c defieiency. withering away, dying!

Diearea since been on ship. Today blead
when went to towlet

Dick hurt *(Then stop touching it!)*

Right ear infliction

Pankeritous

Pulled growns

Human Bite on thumb *(He wasn't kidding;
another sailor deliberately bit him.)*

Check up. And I have a not on my Ass

Ame cavrd in my ey *(What?)*

Jock inch *(I wouldn't brag about that)*

Prisner *(I don't believe that's medically treatable.)*

Fell down stares on my ass

Need a penis (dick) check *(Thanks for clarifying.)*

Urinavee Infection *(Like a humvee infection?)*

Check my hymrode's

Coins on feet *(Put them back in your pocket.)*

Round ball on side of penis *(Basketball injury?)*

Fungs on back and chest

Head cold thort – hard to shalow

Sore heil

Takeing a shit is verry painfull *(Ouch!)*

Would like to see dr. Colon check on my Bronguitis

Blood coming from the erectum

Physical For mess crank. – Get X-Ray on Tail Bone

I'm gonna die! Have the shipyard Flu.

Seaman is yellow *(Those crazy
Navy guys.)*

Gasarithis *(Not a clue.)*

Cracked my gord! *(Laceration on head.)*

Sicle (i.e. Runny nose, watory eyes, small Headache, some chills, slight cough, phlegm)

I have a pain and my chest

Skin earatation

I would like to get some Qual Lotion an have a
Urine Analisis test for any desies *(What?)*

Throughing up diarea
(Talk about your bad breath!)

Noaritis *(Got me.)*

Vensial warts

Around my cruch is eretated

Sore Thorght

Problem breathing Bronqul Passages clogged and
pain on heal of food

I have a groth on my scrodum

Jockage *(A great magazine name!)*

My Back heart'so *(Actually this one is pretty
descriptive)*

Check out Health Records for Ass Medical Officer
(That has to be a tough job.)

I use to have venerolgytis and
I think I got it again
(For God's sake, not again!)

Uron anilizes

Shoulder in joint, Right leg not, would like a X-ray
(I would get that one quickly.)

Towcell *(Not a clue what this is.)*

Spitting up yellow flame *(That has got to hurt!)*

Burning pain in my reactum *(He was
from the reactor department.)*

Hershey squirts

Eskima *(An Alaskan disease?)* ✚

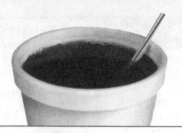

Subj: **Members desperately needed for the XYZ Hospital "Committee" Committee**
Date: Friday, December 14, 2001 12:45:09 AM
From: HR
To: All qualified physicians

A group of 6-8 physicians and administrators to oversee all the other committees and make sure they are truly committed (or should be committed).

Goals include:
1. Developing a plan to oversee the planning strategies
2. Developing a strategy to oversee some of the strategic plans
3. Implementing a core group of competency training goals in order to implement competent training
4. Developing a long-term timeline to make sure all issues are resolved on-time in the long term
5. Drinking coffee

Requirements:*
1. You must enjoy boredom
2. You relish ineffectiveness
3. You like lots of coffee and donuts (or maybe a bagel)
4. You love the sound of your own voice
5. You believe that coming to a conclusion is not really that important and just enjoying the process through discussion is all that matters
6. You have nothing else to do
7. You like to be held or hugged

* You are not an appropriate candidate for this committee if you:
a. Find that you are continually repeating "kill me" to yourself throughout the meeting
b. Possess a "normal" personality
c. Have real friends (Internet pen pals do not count)
d. Like coffee, but understand there is still a limit to everything – even such ambrosia as that of the sweet, sweet nectar squeezed from the magnificent java bean.

Too Personal

After seeing the same female patient for different sexually transmitted diseases over several months, she finally presented to me complaining of a retained tampon. She informed me that although she had been on her period, she had managed to get lucky the night before after a trip to a local bar. Now after her wild night with her new suitor she was afraid the tampon was stuck. After several minutes with the speculum and ring forceps, I managed to extract the offending hygienic product. After its removal I asked her why she hadn't had her partner help her remove the tampon. Her response,

"I didn't know him THAT well!"

Heavy sigh. ✚

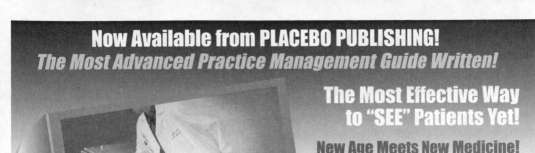

One of the newest crazes in medicine is to use the Internet as a means to make extra money. Online consultation services have been created to offer physicians a chance to use their spare time doing something that comes very natural to them - *answering questions.* Patients pay out of pocket in order to get the doctor's advice on a myriad of topics. *Placebo Journal* wanted to see what this trend is all about and used one of our physicians as a guinea pig. Here's an example from a recent interaction:

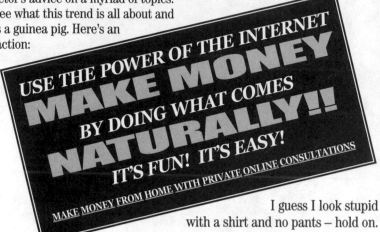

Doctor:
Dr. Parody signing in.

Patient: Hi.

Doctor: Hi, can I help you?

Patient: Yes you can; in so many ways.

Doctor: Alright. Let's get started.

Patient: I would love to.

Doctor: *(after a delay)* What's your question?

Patient: What are you wearing?

Doctor: *(with some confusion):* Well, I am at home at the computer; just got out of my work clothes and into some sweats.

Patient: Are they tight fitting?

Doctor: Well I have put a little weight on . . . hey, wait a minute, this is a medical consultation.

Patient: Can you take them off?

Doctor: Now this is wrong! Well it is a little hot in here . . . ah, what the hell. Hold on a minute (small delay). There, now, what seems to be the problem?

Patient: Are you wearing boxers or briefs?

Doctor: That's really none of your – briefs; they're definitely more comfortable.

Patient: Sounds great, can you take them off?

Doctor: Alright, enough is enough, this really isn't the point of a medical consultation – wait while I shut the door first.

Patient: Now take all your clothes off.

Doctor: Well that seems like a little much; my wife is in the next room.

I guess I look stupid with a shirt and no pants – hold on.

Patient: Do you have any lotion?

Doctor: You mean like a cortisone cream or something?

Patient: No, not a damn cortisone cream! Lotion or oil?

Doctor: I have butter.

Patient: Butter? That's sick.

Doctor: Well, this was supposed to be a medical consultation.

Patient: Then why do you have butter?

Doctor: Does it really matter? I get lonely sometimes.

Patient: Forget it, I'm chatting with some-one else; you're one sick bast*rd.

Doctor: No – don't go; I'm still here. *Come back!!* What are you wearing? I have bananas here too!!

As you can see, this area of medical consultation looks very promising. In fact, our Dr. Parody has been trying to find this patient continually for the last month. We see exciting things for the future of this new medium and look forward to the day when it adds to our ability to help patients. ✚

This person has a problem. Their upper denture plate is not where it should be . . .

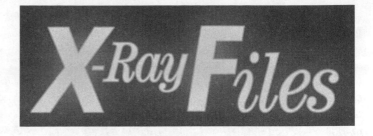

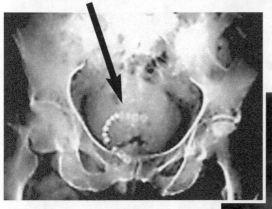

. . . and could use ideas on how to continue good oral hygiene.

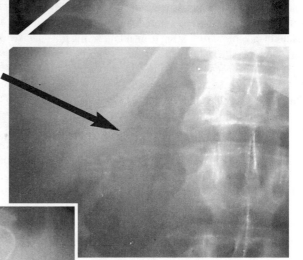

These people might have a solution.

Swallow your toothbrush.
(Just don't get it caught in your esophagus, like this!)

Swallow your toothbrush harder.
(Gets it all the way down to your stomach, like this!)

Or, you could try going at it another way.
(Not like this, remove the toothbrush holder first for better oral hygiene.)

We are not here to knock the occupation of the pharmaceutical representative. They can help in a many situations and they do have a job to do. Many of them are young and right out of college. Stepping into the real world after being brainwashed by their companies just sets them up to get their asses ripped by overworked physicians. Sure it is easy to get rid of them from your office. You could have a "No Rep Policy." You could put up hurdles that they could never overcome. You could just be rude and vicious. We do not believe in these techniques. *Why be a jerk when you can have some fun?* So the question is: how can you get rid of some reps without being mean or resorting to violence? Here are five easy and fun ways:

5 EFFECTIVE TECHNIQUES TO HELP YOU COMMUNICATE WITH PHARMACEUTICAL REPRESENTATIVES

(WITHOUT BEING MEAN OR RESORTING TO VIOLENCE)

1 The "Three-Year-Old" Technique

How many times do you get stuck in a conversation with a drug rep that you cannot get out of? You want to be nice (*you really do*), but they keep pushing. You want to give them a quick thanks, but with verbal gymnastics you are caught in a debate about minutia. You can't remember studies. You can't even remember your spouse's name because you're busting your hump trying to see a full schedule of patients.

The "Three-Year-Old" Technique is a metaphor for talking to a little child. Recently, my daughter was explaining some story about being at a big slide and running around. I tried to tell her that I wasn't sure it was me that was there.

"Remember, Dad?" she said.

"No, I can't remember," I responded.

"We had fun at the place."

"I am not sure. What was it about?"

She would scream back that it was a big slide and there were balloons. I said, *"Honey, maybe Mommy was with you but I was at work or something."* The more I debated the more she got upset and dug her feet in.

Then I said, *"Oh, you mean the big slide? With all the balloons?"* She smiled and said, *"Yeah, remember?"* I said that I did and we changed the subject without any more fuss.

Now here is a typical interaction with a pharmaceutical representative that sets you up for failure: *"Doctor, remember the last time we spoke and I gave you that article?"*

98

"No, I can't remember."

"Well I left it on your desk."

"I am not sure. What was it about?"

"It was about how our medication is more efficacious than our competition's medication."

"But all the drugs in that class of medication are basically the same."

"That's not true. Remember that our medication has fewer side effects and almost 2 percent more drop in systolic blood pressure than the others."

"Is that really significant?"

"If you remember, that article stated . . ."

In the above conversation, you may be stuck losing precious minutes of your life whereupon cutting your own jugular may be your only viable option. By using the "Three-Year-Old" Technique you can make this interaction quick and painless. Let's see that same conversation again:

"Doctor, remember the last time we spoke and I gave you that article?"

"Yes."

"What did you think about the drop in blood pressure and the fewer side effects?"

*"Oh, you mean lower blood pressure (**the big slide**)? With the fewer side effects (**all the balloons**)?"*

"Yeah, remember?" I said that I did and we changed the subject without anymore fuss.

2 Making Irritable Bowel Syndrome Your Friend

Don't let this demon of a disease be your enemy anymore. Use it to your advantage when you see a pharmaceutical representative. Every time you see one, start to cramp. Bend over and shake. Rub your side. How many times have you held back your flatulent urge anyway? With this technique, you let it rip! Wiggle and wriggle and then excuse yourself to go to the bathroom. Just like you can't prove your patients have anything real, neither can the drug reps. After a while you will have trained yourself to just point to the bathroom as soon as you see the rep and they will just know where you are headed (*even if it is a small white lie*). Even better, you can start getting creative. You can buy a can of "Fart Spray" at the local magic shop and spray it in your office. Invite the drug rep to come in and really try to get into a deep conversation. Watch them squirm. This technique will be so much fun that you will look forward to the cohort of detailers that comes your way. Since they all know each other, the word will spread quickly and they will hate having to see you because you either will be running to the bathroom or embarrassing them. Save your best tricks for when their boss comes in with them. The beauty of this whole technique is that if you actually prescribe enough of their drug they are forced to come see you.

Now who is bothering whom?

3 Pretend You Are a Mime

Everyone hates mimes.

4 Show Them Your Beautiful Mind

Schizophrenia is a terrible disease and not something to joke about. It is, however, very effective in making pharmaceutical reps leave. Next time one of them comes in, thank them for bringing their "stuff." Bring them aside and ask if they were followed to your office. Question why they know your "numbers." Baffle them with remarks like, *"I have been hoarding your medicine at home in case the invasion occurs. Can you send more directly to my house?"* You need to be subtle and not laugh or let them know you are joking.

When they ask if you are putting them on, you need to stand your ground and say things like, *"So I guess you are on their side? They got to you and you don't even know it"* or *"You are not fooling me, Lord Kaslov. Maybe we need to settle this once and for all."* Then just walk away slowly staring at them the whole time. Don't smile. Immediately knock on the door of the next patient's room and walk in. Prep your staff to tell the rep that you are having some "problems" and I guarantee they will never come back to talk to you again.

5 Ask Them Out

This sounds very sick and perverted, but it works. Even if they are the same sex as you, just do it. Even if you are married and are forty years older than them, just do it. Nothing will make them more uncomfortable than that. If you are going to ask them out, be creative. Tempt them with a date to a topless bar. Ask them, *"Have you ever been to a satanic church?"* See if they want to go for a trip to the nursing home to see your grandmother. Inquire whether they want to join you in a high colonic. If for any reason, a drug rep says yes, take them to the mall and shop *Victoria's Secret* – for about an hour. If they are still with you, pick up a sexy piece of lingerie and ask the worker, *"You think this will fit my mother?"* **This last part is foolproof.**

We hope you use these techniques in order to enjoy your interactions with pharmaceutical representatives. Like the mail, this sales force will never stop coming. Like stepping on cockroaches while standing on a mattress, you can push as hard as you'd like, but you are never going to kill them. Instead of fighting hard and stressing yourself out, use the above recommendations to make your life a little happier. ✚

This is the strange but true tale of an extraordinarily obese middle-aged woman whom we will call Bertha. My partner admitted Bertha to the ICU for hypoxia (a lack of oxygen) and hyercapnea (an increase in carbon dioxide, meaning she wasn't breathing well) after she exhibited signs of altered consciousness at home. She was enormous at over 400 lbs. *This was a big woman.* She responded to the usual modalities and she was transferred to a general medical bed. There was something odd about Bertha. She would always lie on her side, never supine. She was stabilized and discharge to home was ordered. When the EMT people attempted to place her supine on a stretcher – she immediately syncopated and went into V-tach. A code ensued, and of course I was on call to administer aid. She miraculously responded to the "family joules" (getting shocked) and epinephrine and regained consciousness when placed back in bed on her side.

So, another course of ICU monitoring was initiated, she stabilized and went again to the general medical floor. The day of reckoning approached (i.e., her new day of discharge). Of course I was in charge again. I thought, how bizarre! What is the mechanism of her postural instability – acute hypoxia from monstrous mammary tissue causing lung compression or *the sheer terror she must have had of the gurney shattering to smithereens after her weight was placed on it!*

The afternoon came and I thought I was ready. A team of four EMT workers were prepared; they brought their biggest stretcher. I was there to lend assistance along with at least three other nurses and the patient's son. We successfully placed her on the stretcher lying

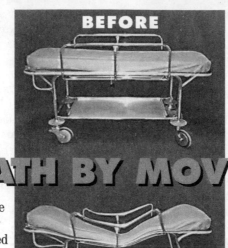

BEFORE

DEATH BY MOVING

AFTER?

slightly on her side. She was frightened but cooperating. Her vitals remained stable. Her pannus (folds of abdominal fat) hung over the seemingly narrow stretcher like a wet sponge. *I thought the aluminum frame of the gurney would collapse under the weight of our pitiful rider as it squealed down the aisle with the train of seven health care workers.*

As the entourage reached the hospital entrance I took a right into the doctor's lounge, proud of my heroic accomplishment. Breathing a sigh of relief, I reassured my team I would stay on the premises until they drove off into the sunset. I congratulated myself on a job well done, certainly more conscientious than any of my partners could've performed. Then I heard the ominous *"Code Blue! Code Blue!"* over the P.A. followed by my beeper buzzing. My heart sank as my pride bubble burst. She went unconscious and coded just before the EMT people were going to shut the door of the ambulance! This time she didn't survive the code, hence the title of this article.

EPILOGUE: Her remains were so voluminous the hospital morgue didn't have the capacity to store her! Later I spoke with the funeral director who was to receive her remains in a capped pick-up truck. He told me that it was common knowledge that Bertha had brought illness onto herself from self-destructive eating habits and this infamous episode would not surprise her neighbors.

Remember Bertha when counseling your patients on the consequences of obesity. Tell them if they won't bridle their passion for eating, the last thing they'll taste is . . .

DEATH BY MOVING

✚

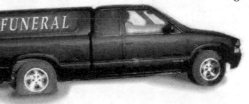

FUNERAL

MY FAVORITE MUNCHAUSEN

CLIPPING

Mary was 37 and needed her knee done. Like many athletes, getting an arthroscopy was important so that she could get back to her favorite activities. The surgery was initially hailed as a success as the right knee went under arthroscopy and a lateral release for her chronic knee pain. *Unfortunately, things turned for the worse soon thereafter.*

It seems a synovial fistula (draining hole in her knee) developed at the site where one of the portals of the arthroscope had gone through. The physicians acted quickly by placing her knee in a cast and giving her antibiotics. What was felt to be another success (as the fistula did heal) was met with failure again. On three other occasions, Mary had breakdown of her knee with more drainage at the site. The doctors pushed hard to get Mary to be compliant with more hospital admissions for bed rest and plaster cast immobilization.

This was not to be.

During the next four months after the surgery and failure after failure, poor Mary agreed to have another surgery to repair the draining fistula. This time, however, our heroes got smarter and during the operation they really explored the knee for a cause of the problem.

Wouldn't you know it; a straightened paper-clip attached to a piece of string was found and removed.

Now how the hell did that get in there?

Mary went on to have long-term antibiotics as her knee was now septic. Upon asking her where the clip came from, Mary turned ugly. She was defensive and insisted that somehow the clip was put in there by the surgeon. The surgeon disagreed, as placing paper clips attached to a string is not standard of care, even for some of the worst HMOs.

Finally, the struggle ended when Mary confessed her sins to a sympathetic nurse. She said she put the paper clip into the wound to block the hole so that she could go scuba diving. There was one problem with this story, however. Mary had never even scuba dived before. Maybe it is similar to that joke when a patient asks a physician, *"After my surgery can I play the piano?"* The surgeon responds, *"Sure, are you any good?"* whereupon the patient responds, *"I've never tried."*

Mary is still receiving psychiatric treatment to this day. ✚

This story was liberally embellished from: J.R. Coll. Surg. Edinb. *42, Aug. 1997, 252-53.*

POWER LUNCH

One day when I was running behind (*and what day was I not?*), I only had one pregnant patient left to see. Being a nice boss I sent my office staff out to lunch. This 18-week primip (first pregnancy) had been having some significant nausea and vomiting earlier in her pregnancy, so I asked how she had been feeling lately. Almost as soon as she responded *"Much better!"* she proceeded to have projectile vomiting (*pizza with the works*) all over me, the exam table, the counter and the carpet. None of the vomit got on her, of course, which is one of the true hidden pluses of projectile vomiting.

After she and her husband left (*as she declared that she now felt "Even better!"*), it dawned on me that with no office staff around to help clean up, Yours Truly was going to have to clean it all up.

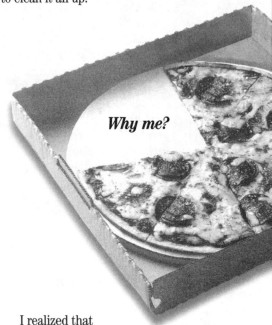

Why me?

I realized that I had had a very helpful and valuable experience. Now when I lay in bed at night and think about the day, no matter how bad it had been, I say to myself, *"Well, at least no one threw up on me today!"* And then I think about ordering a pizza.

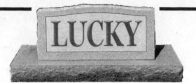

LUCKY

TALES FROM COLLEGE HEALTH

I work at a college health clinic at a large East Coast university. I recently saw a local kid, a commuter student, for a sinus problem. He'd had a sinus infection about a month ago and was still having symptoms.

"What symptoms did you have?"

"Well, I had a sinus infection, but it got treated, and now I just have some symptoms left."

"What did your doctor treat you with?"

"Weelll . . .[sheepish look] *I took some old antibiotics that were left over. My mom said it was okay."*

"What did you take?"

"It was cephalexin, I think."

"How much did you take? What was the dose?"

"Weelll . . . [sheepish look] *I'm not sure. I mean, it wasn't my prescription . . .* [more sheepish look] *it was my dog's. I mean, my mom said it was the same stuff that a people doctor would prescribe . . ."*

"How many times a day were they for?"

"They were supposed to be twice a day, so I just took them once a day to be safe." ("To be safe" being a relative term at this point.) Hmmm. I don't know why I asked, maybe to guesstimate the dose.

"How big is your dog?"

"Oh, about 100 pounds."

"What is he, a Newfie? A St. Bernard?"

"No, he's a yellow lab."

"I guess he's a big one." Then I got a judgmental look on my face. *"Look, I'm not so concerned that you're taking old antibiotics, but I AM concerned that your dog didn't get HIS full treatment course."*

"Weelll . . . [sheepish look] *he actually passed on a while ago. These were just left over."*

So they didn't even help the dog, I thought. ✚

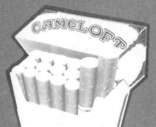
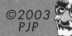

FLATUS MAXIMUS

There is a unique human condition which has afflicted us all, yet doesn't merit research dollars or articles in medical journals. It is known by a variety of names the world over, but scientific nomenclature favors the term *"flatulence."* Indeed, there are legions of quietly distressed sufferers of this malady. Who among us has not experienced the occasional indignity of the escape of an errant passage of methane fumes, then glanced furtively around to see if anyone has noticed? Who in primary care or gastroenterology has not had a patient shame-facedly inquire about what they can do for their socially challenging *"gas"* problem? Many of my patients confess this most embarrassing secret to me, and all this time I thought it was just me so afflicted.

I have had a wealth of personal experience with this topic. *Who hasn't?* But I am the unlikely inheritor of what my mother refers to as the *"Choury bowels,"* and my family can trace its flatulent past to nineteenth-century French ancestors.

Being thus accursed with this ignominious family trait, I had my first public experience with gas as an innocent sixth-grader. On this particular day, I had feasted on a large portion of my mother's greasy hashed-browns for lunch, then went to my piano club recital. I was seated in the audience listening to a fellow student perform when I suddenly noticed a rumbling in my stomach. Then a loud gust trumpeted from me and echoed off the fine acoustics of the recital hall.

I was horrified!

Somehow everyone managed to pretend they heard nothing. The pianist kept playing. Several minutes later, the unthinkable happened again. My colon threatened to erupt once more. I gritted my teeth and every muscle in my body, all to no avail. Another high decibel blast mingled with the lyrical notes of the Hadyn sonata. This was just too much for my musical grade-school colleagues to overlook. A chorus of snickers threatened to distract the performer. Then the two girls in front of me nearly collapsed on each other, shoulders shaking with convulsive laughter. I wanted desperately to slither out of the room. Instead, in my mortified state I sat rigid, stared straight ahead past the giggling girls and tried to pretend that those unmistakable noises did not emanate from me.

Somehow I gained better control of myself and survived the remainder of my adolescence unscathed by such improprieties. In fact, it wasn't until my third year of medical school that I committed another serious error in judgment. I had undergone a rather depressing dateless spell for several years when I was invited out by a fellow medical student. I was so excited I even purchased a new outfit for the rare event. This was a departure from my usual medical school thrift, characterized by spartan budget and a steady diet of cheap canned goods. The night before the big date, I made the spectacularly regrettable choice of consuming an entire can of baked beans for dinner. The following afternoon, I was in a panic upon realizing that an inferno was raging in my abdomen and showed no signs of abating. I overdosed myself with antacids but they were pitifully poor protection against the gas which silently torpedoed from me. After my date picked me up I managed to control the situation until we arrived at the restaurant. But once we started eating, I could no longer stifle my gastrocolic reflex. *Soon a particularly pungent cloud floated about me.* I was aghast at the realization that my date could hardly mistake the odor, but he mercifully feigned ignorance of the whole malodorous affair. I tried to keep my distance from him and made several extended trips to the bathroom, all without success. As the evening closed on my all-time date disaster and he dropped me off at my apartment door, I could scarcely believe my ears as I heard him ask if he could take me out again.

He was truly a brave soul.

Not surprisingly, surviving the remainder of medical school proved to be a challenge for me. Yes, the academics were bad enough, but I also had to endure long rounds with my medical teams. Rounds held in closed conference rooms were the worst. I would secretly palm an antacid tablet in my pocket, then pop it into my mouth. *I'd chew slowly, hoping no one would ask me a question while I had a mouthful of chalk.* Walking rounds were less hazardous, but still presented a challenge at times. While on my medicine rotation, I ate peanut M&M's for dinner every night, not yet realizing that peanuts were a prime gas producer for me. One day on afternoon walking rounds, I felt the familiar borborygmi and I just had to silently let one fly. *Much to my horror, the smell was terrible and traveled quickly.* I stole a sidelong glance at my fellow med students. Everyone was standing in a semicircle attentively listening to our senior resident. As the foul odor disseminated amongst our team, it triggered a cascade of reactions. First the stifled snickers and finger pointing began. Then the three other third-year students moved en masse across the circle away from Steve, the only fourth-year student. Poor

Steve stood alone, facing the crowd who had deemed it too noxious to stand next to him. He was publicly convicted of the malodorous deed while I let him take the blame and laughed along with the others.

But not everyone was fooled.

As rounds disintegrated into junior high league jostling, my senior resident aimed a withering glare at me.

Oh God, he knew it was really me!

Still the coward, I pretended not to notice and meekly rejoined my team at the next patient's room.

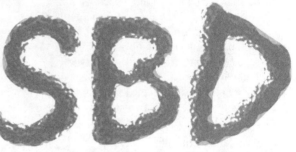

After several more years of less harrowing experiences, I finally learned which foods to avoid before important dates, long hours of lecture, and later, extended office hours. I found industrial strength simethicone at the drugstore and dosed myself with it when necessary. Completion of my residency brought two welcome surprises with it. The first was that my gastrointestinal distress diminished with the decline of stressors in my life. The second was that I met a handsome Air Force officer shortly thereafter. It wasn't until almost a year later that I discovered that my prospective groom suffered a lifelong disability – congenital anosmia.

The man of my dreams had no sense of smell!

It was truly a match made in olfactory heaven. We were married soon after and now await the arrival of yet another generation of children with colicky, flatulent *"Choury bowels."* ✚

A Problem Patient Comes and Goes

She was a new patient and I had not previously met her. After I entered the exam room and gave my customary greeting and introduction, she declared, *"I'm a manic-depressive, adult attention deficit disorder, borderline personality."* Well, this is going to be interesting, I thought to myself. Yes, indeed.

After a rather elaborate history had been taken, I began the physical examination. The first thing that seemed odd occurred when I began the examination of her heart. As was customary (with respect to the average patient's modesty), I kept her front covered as I placed my stethoscope under her gown to lay it over the usual listening sites. This time, however, I got hung up on a chain that seemed suspended between her breasts, although she was supine at the time. After I disentangled my stethoscope and finished the cardiac exam, the mystery of the chain was solved. Like a main cable crossing the center span of a suspension bridge, her bridged towers were represented by (pierced) nipple rings on top of silicon foundations and the chain was strung across them. My first thought was, *"OUCH, that must have hurt."* Seeing my obvious grimace, she assured me that it hadn't been that bad, and the purpose of the arrangement was to enhance (sexual) pleasure when the chain was pulled.

"OK now, let's quickly move on to the rest of the exam," I thought. Nearing the completion of the exam, I felt relieved that she was seeing a gynecologist and thus didn't need to be examined by me in that regard. *Alas, such was not the case.* She hesitantly stated that she had a problem that she needed my opinion about. *"Oh, what the hell - you've seen it all anyway,"* and proceeded to yank the material of her short-shorts aside to expose her genitalia, complete with a clitoral ring. ***Did I know how to take the ring off?*** It was at this point that I wondered if we could get a security buzzer for the exam rooms like the bank tellers have. The story continues. It seemed that her husband got sort of *"chewed up"* the last time they had sex (in spite of their

use of "Slick" brand personal lubricant), and so he wanted the ring removed. Observing the ring from a respectable distance, I demurred, stating it was way out of my area of expertise and as she was the first patient I had ever seen with such jewelry. I suggested that whoever had put it in would surely be able to remove it. If not that person, then perhaps her gynecologist could be of assistance. ***The bottom line was that it wasn't going to be me.*** I then excused myself (*escaped!*) while she dressed.

After that first visit, her subsequent visits always made me a little uneasy as I never knew what to expect. One time she came in and wanted me to run every test for VD on her that I could. She suspected her husband of being unfaithful and eventually they did get divorced, but not before she took her revenge. One time she tried to show my office staff a photo she found in her house of an unclearly identified male in an aroused state (*"I know it's my husband because I recognize the lamp next to him"*). Another time she claimed to have sent a postcard to his new location (living with relatives out of state), writing on it that he had better get himself checked for VD (even though all her tests had come back normal). It was at this time that I told her that her behavior wasn't appropriate and she needed to "move on." She took my advice literally and moved to another county. When the request for a copy of her medical records arrived from her new doctor, I felt a wave of relief sweep over me. It was none too soon, for on our last visit she put me in the dilemma of having to choose between her short-term impulses and the opposing principle of what was best for her (*and society*) in the long run: she complained about her loss of sexual desire and what could be done about it? ✚

EDITOR'S NOTE: *Thanks for sharing about your "problem" patient. You should have told her about your lack of desire . . . lack of desire to see her. Or you could have put the clitoral ring back in!*

HAIRPIN CURVE

My wife (we'll call her Amy), a wonderfully competent board certified and usually very empathic psychiatrist, escorted the tearful, middle-aged woman out of her office to have her rescheduled and get her some medication samples.

When she brought her into her office for the psychiatric interview, she nestled back into her chair with pen at poise – her office emanating that low, "womb-like" comfort lighting. During the interview, Amy thought the patient had a rather unusual hairpin of sorts in place above her forehead, but was riveted by the tale of loss and sadness and focused on trying to help her through this major depression.

Now, interview complete, in the full fluorescent light of the main office, as the patient approached the scheduling desk, our receptionist remarked, *"So, who's your friend?"* The patient looked perplexed and then Amy turned around and saw the *"hairpin"* in all its glory.

It seems that the patient had walked out of her home, in a hurry to get to her appointment, and passed through some type of spiderweb. Now, embedded in her hair spray-hardened hair, was the brittle, but large carcass of a thoroughly deceased Japanese beetle embraced by the tender silken threads of the web.

Amy just absolutely lost it – she tried not to laugh but before she knew what was happening she was laughing so hard she was crying. Now, usually, the psychiatrist doesn't laugh out loud after having just spent an hour with a tearful, depressed patient, but Amy could not help herself. To no one's surprise, the patient never returned. ✚

A BAD ITCH

I was trained in Syria and did my residency in the United States. This story happened two months after the 9/11 tragedy.

A young woman came to see me on a Monday afternoon. Apparently on Saturday, she ate seafood (some shrimp and what have you). A few hours later she developed a rash with severe itching. In the emergency room, our friend was given a shot for the reaction and told to follow up with me. Nothing remarkable was found on my exam, but she was still having the itch.

After we finished our discussion, I made a decision and said, *"Madam, I am going to give you some Atarax."*

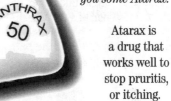

Atarax is a drug that works well to stop pruritis, or itching.

Unfortunately, the patient didn't truly understand what I said. With a frightened look on her face she screamed, **"No, sir, do not give me ANTHRAX, I don't want that!"**

The lesson here is to always be careful with your pronunciation especially if you have a foreign accent.

✚

A FAMILY DOC IN THE LAND OF THE AMISH

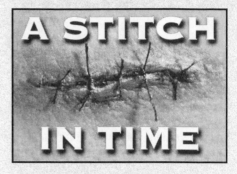

A STITCH IN TIME

An Amish man came in with a chief complaint of having his *"right ear blocked for two years."* He had a big piece of cotton stuck in the ear after trying "sweet oil" and other natural remedies. I checked the ear and it was indeed packed with cotton and wax. After my nurse did extensive lavage, I rechecked the canal and found it clear. As I handed him the bill he said, *"Doctor, can I have my cotton ball back?"* I handed it to him and asked, *"What do you want it for?"* He responded, *"Well, everything is so loud now."* Guess I'll be seeing him back in a couple of years.

Another time I came in after hours on a weekend to sew up a seven-year-old Amish child. He had cut himself in the forehead playing with sharp and dangerous farm implements. The father brought him along with three other children. I soon figured out that the *"yes, we are patients in your practice"* over the phone actually meant *"we go to the other doc up the road, but he won't come in on weekends."* With a sigh, I had the father fill out the patient information sheet while I set up the suture tray.

I looked at the sheet and said, *"Okay . . . Jacob, hop up on the table and let's take a look."* This kid was incredibly stoic. Not a flinch when I said, *"Okay, Jacob, now you'll feel a bee sting as I numb you up."* Jacob never moved a muscle or said a word. I fixed him without a problem and told dad to call the office for a suture removal appointment in five days.

Seventeen days later, Mom brings him back in. The front desk can't find his chart anywhere. After ten minutes of searching in vain, I tell my staff to just put him in a room. I figured I would take his sutures out and find the chart later. As I am struggling to extract my now completely buried handiwork from his forehead (he's as stoic and wordless as ever), I say, *"Sorry, Jacob, I know that this may hurt a little . . ."*

Mom cuts me off and with a big smile says, *"Oh! It wondered me why you didn't find the record of him! This is Amos, not Jacob. My husband always gets them mixed!"* ✚

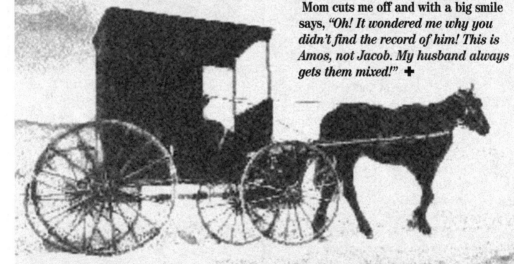

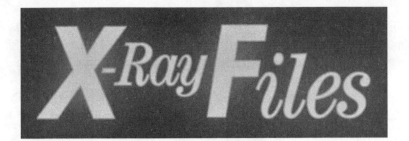

He did.

She did.

The remote was removed under general anesthesia.

I remember having a case of a mini-Munchausen about eight years ago. I did a Bier Block (a type of local anesthesia) on a lady for hand surgery. I had to give her a social dose of Versed for her severe anxiety. We took her to the Recovery Room, where we noted she was unconscious. Then she started posturing in a weird paralyzed sort of position. I thought maybe she got walloped with a big slug of IV lidocaine when we let the tourniquet down – even though we did it slowly and watched her in the OR before we went to Recovery. I started treating for local anesthetic overdose.

STRIKE A POSE

After thirty minutes she was still posturing and unconscious. I called for a stat neurological consult. The guy walks in, lifts her hand up in the air and lets go . . . and her hand stays up! He turns to me and says, *"She's awake"* and walks out.

I go running down the hall after him. He tells me that holding her hand up like that is a voluntary movement and he's going back to the office.

Man, it never occurred to me!
I used to do that trick in the ER holding the hand over the face and dropping it. Truly unconscious people will hit themselves in the face – if you let the hand actually fall that far – whereas fakers will always have the hand drop off to the side.
But I never saw the hand stay in the air.
Anyway, I go out to face her husband. He asks if he can see her. I take him to the recovery room, he looks at her, shrugs his shoulders, and says,

She does that all the time."
I couldn't believe it!
Finally he tells me she sees a shrink. I call the psychiatrist and he goes ballistic. Apparently, this lady had a bad "incident" in the hospital as a child after a tonsillectomy and keeps having surgery. The unconsciousness is a conversion reaction.
Over the next year I saw her in pre-op two more times and had to call her shrink and the surgeon each time to get the procedure canceled.

Who says we never learn.
I bet this young lady keeps torturing other anesthesiologists today. ✛

He
didn't
have
a job.

He didn't have
a dime.

Bill Millionaire
had nothing
until . . .
he sued
his doctor
for
malpractice.

BILL MILLIONAIRE.
*It's the funniest
reality television show yet.*

Here's the twist.
Bill Millionaire has a little secret.
Shhh, don't tell anyone.
Bill Millionaire isn't even sick!

Watch Bill Millionaire get
three different lawyers
to salivate over his case.

See him fool three
"specialists" into
believing he really is ill.

Observe empathetic
jurors as they fall for
Bill's deception and
hand out millions for
pain and suffering.

BILL MILLIONAIRE

**BILL MILLIONAIRE.
The joke is on us and
we're all paying for it!**

Only on

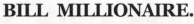

POX TV

*The only station
that would sell
its kidney for
better ratings.*

SCOOBY SNACK

A man cut off his penis to spite his girlfriend and said that it was left on the kitchen floor. The rescue squad was sent back to retrieve it with the possibility of reattaching the member. When they got there they found that the dog had eaten it. ✚

TRUE ANECDOTES

An aerospace engineer came in with five days of rectal bleeding. He saved all of his used toilet paper and brought it in to the exam in a plastic bag in case the doc wanted to see it.

There are some things even a $15 co-pay won't cover.

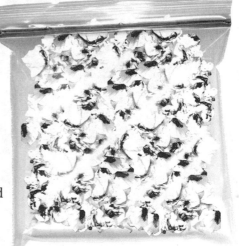

A lady who kept trying to kill herself was found unconscious with her head in the oven. Paramedics called in to the ER stated that she had carbon monoxide poisoning because of her bright red face. Trouble was, only her face was red.

Diagnosis: drug overdose followed by placing head in an electric oven, causing first-degree burns.

A patient today who is a total train wreck with arachnoiditis (inflammation of the spine) and spinal stenosis (narrowing of the spinal cord) now with a failed back. He asked me for a script for Viagra. I was blown away. *Who would he be having sex with? And how?* He was going to Mexico for a funeral the next day. He told me, *"Doc, I haven't had sex in two years, I'm going to Mexico tomorrow and I'm going to get laid even if I have to get AIDS."*

112

**We don't stand a chance.
The patients are winning. ✚**

A TRUE DIAGNOSIS

I was called to do an epidural on a young lady having her second child. This expectant mother was all of thirteen. Although this young girl was in tremendous pain, both she and her 30-year-old mother were able to answer my questions regarding her medical history. There wasn't much to it until I asked her what medicines she was taking at home. She replied,

"Nothing but that Adderal. That's because I'm hyperactive."

"I'll say!"

jumped out of my mouth before I could think. The patient didn't respond but the 30-year-old grandmother, OB nurse, and I had a great laugh.✚

EDITOR'S NOTE - It's not easy biting your tongue. I might have said something more enlightening like *"At this rate you'll be post-menopausal by age nineteen."*

felt so good.

GIRLS JUST WANNA HAVE FUN

TROUBLE

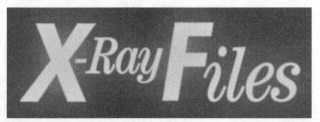

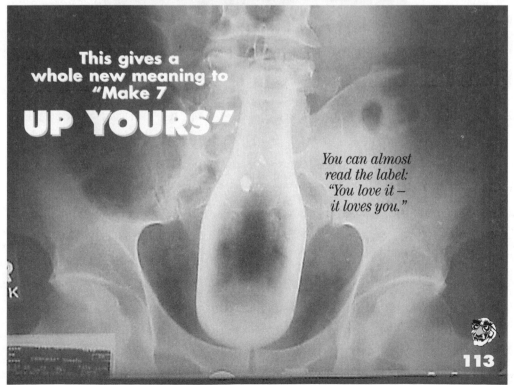

This gives a whole new meaning to "Make 7

UP YOURS"

You can almost read the label: "You love it — it loves you."

MY FAVORITE
MUNCHAUSEN

These Munchausens are a couple of kooky "diabetics" who don't know each other but have a heck of a lot in common.

Sarah was a 27-year-old woman who complained of terrible left groin pain. No one was able to define what the problem was. She eventually was sent to an endocrinologist because of her history of diabetes. It seems she had had this disease since age thirteen. *"Strange, but she only acquired diabetes during this past year?"* he thought.

Gertrude was 18 years of age and she too had diabetes. Her primary care doctor thought that she would need the help of a specialist (the same endocrinologist). The weird thing about Gerty was that she only consulted her family doctor once about the need for insulin and *whoosh*, she was whisked away to the specialist. She did have high blood sugar readings on her home monitor; however, and had problems with polyuria (urinating all the time) and polydipsia (drinking all the time).

Sarah had an immense past medical history for such a young girl. She had a hysterectomy for heavy menstrual bleeding, a laparoscopy for chronic abdominal pain and surgery to remove a malignant tumor from her arm (no record could be found on that one).

Gertrude had some interesting medical problems as well. Another hospital had found that she had psychogenic polydipsia. In other words, she would drink water to excess and this would

INSULIN-CRAVIN'
SWEET TEETH

make her physically ill. Upon further inspection, Sarah also had been diagnosed with psychogenic polydipsia in the past. *What was going on here?*

The plot thickens. Sarah's husband had type I diabetes and needed insulin. Gerty's boyfriend also had type I diabetes and needed insulin. *Here is the kicker.* Both were found to have normal glucose testing while being hospitalized! There were no abnormally high levels found on regular finger sticks. No abnormalities on glycohemoglobin testing. There were no abnormalities on oral glucose testing. Our endocrinologist got wise and brought in another specialist. *Wouldn't you know it, both Sarah and Gertrude were labeled as Munchausens by the same psychiatrist.* Our physician hero picked up both Sarah and Gerty because he was able to hospitalize them. This was an advantage the primary care doctors didn't have. In a contained environment and with a good eye *(as well as suspicion)*, physicians everywhere have a chance to spot one of these rare Munchies.

No, Sarah and Gerty were not the same person nor did they know each other. *Was their modus operandi of shooting their significant others' insulin a coincidence?* Were their similar histories a "twilight zone" theme? We don't know the answer to these questions. What we do know is that there are probably more sweethearts like Sarah and Gertrude out there and they are coming your way. ✚

This story was liberally embellished from: Aust NZ J Med *1998; 28.*

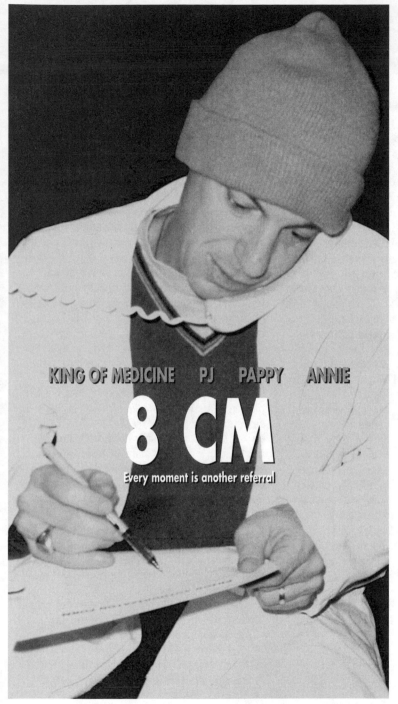

KING OF MEDICINE   PJ   PAPPY   ANNIE

8 CM

Every moment is another referral

MOVIE REVIEW

The only film that shows how to keep medicine real.

Experience a young man's journey from an honor student in an upper-class neighborhood to become a doctor in an upper-class neighborhood.

See him struggle with his mother's guilt . . . "Your grandfather was a doctor. Your father was a doctor. How can you not be a doctor?"

Watch "Dougy from the Block" struggle with an addiction to caffeine and very jealous classmates to become the King of Medicine.

See him drop his rap on a HMO representative trying to block a dermatological referral for an 8 cm malignant skin lesion.

See Dr. Doug take on this procedure himself. Without the experience. Without the right equipment.

"You only got one lidocaine shot, do not miss your chance to sew."

"Incredible. This may actually inspire others to do something. I was kidding. Not really."
Bill Osler, *Tenesmus Gazette*

Polyp and Fissure says, "Two upgoing Babinskis!"

115

These types of patients all do the same thing because they have the same motive.
My hat goes off to the physician who had to live through the hell.

I am a psychiatrist. I was working in a hospital in NYC, in the outpatient mental health clinic. Upon arrival, I inherited a caseload of many patients from my overloaded peers, usually without getting any details or warnings about the patients. Everyone was just too busy for a "sign-out" of patients.

One of the patients was "Bonnie," a 38-year-old black female who was on Klonopin for her "Generalized Anxiety Disorder." She would never keep her monthly scheduled appointments, but would come in now and then and demand to be seen on the spot. More specifically, she would come to my office and bang on my door, and insist on being seen right away. She often claimed she'd *"lost her Klonopin"* (a controlled substance, a benzodiazepine). This is a frequent occurrence, because Klonopin can be abused, taken excessively, or even sold in the street (*for $3 a pill!*). Naturally, psychiatrists are hesitant about replacing a prescription. The first time she *"lost"* her bottle (*"I left it on the bus"*) my supervisor and I spoke and we decided to give her a week's worth, with no refills. Bonnie came back in three days saying she *"had dropped them down the sink accidentally."* Her attitude was belligerent and bullying. This time I refused to refill it. She got angry and left yelling at me as she walked away. Subsequently, Bonnie went to her therapist and said I had been *"abusive to her."*

Twenty minutes later she opened my office door (*I should have kept it locked*), strode up to my desk and brought her fist down on my forehead. She ran out of the clinic. A welt immediately appeared on my forehead. I was sent down to the ER, given Tylenol and some ice for my head.

I asked my family if I should press charges. They said, *"Nah, what can you do, she's mentally ill."* The next week at work, my boss called me in; *"A detective came here looking for you."* He'd left a number, which I called. He told me that on the day the patient punched me, she'd gone to the local precinct and filed a complaint stating that I had *"hit her on the head with a staple gun."* I had to consult with a lawyer (big bucks!) who accompanied me down to the precinct to straighten this out.

A month later, the patient's caseworker admitted to me that the patient had assaulted the doctor who had previously covered this patient. One day this patient barged into her office while she was with another patient. Bonnie (my assailant) demanded to be seen right away. When the doctor asked her to wait outside, she picked up an umbrella and hit the doctor over the head with it, then took the umbrella and swept all the charts off the doctor's desk onto the floor. All the warning signs and the pattern of behavior were there. Then I arrived on the job – and the patient was transferred to me, without any warnings from this doctor or the caseworker.

I asked my boss what we could do about this patient. He said we *"should all meet with her and agree to a verbal contract that would set limits on her behavior."* He sent her a letter inviting her to such a meeting, but she never came in. A secretary in the front office was the only one who comforted me. She said *"There's no excuse for that patient hitting you. Even mental illness is no excuse."*

Thank you, voice of sanity.

Needless to say, I changed jobs soon thereafter. The clinic director wrote her a letter stating she was not to return to the clinic and her chart was being closed. She could, however, get help at other clinics in the area and listed the names and phone numbers of those three other centers. Wouldn't you know it but one of those clinics was where I worked at part-time! (*The idiot hadn't asked me where else I worked!*)

Luckily, I never saw the patient, or her fist, again. ✚

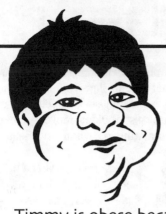

The
Timmy Fund

Timmy is sedentary because television has made him that way.

Timmy is obese because the fast food industry addicted him to their product.

Timmy drinks a case of beer a day because he is bored.

Timmy smokes three packs of cigarettes before noon because the tobacco companies make him do it.

Timmy is on disability because he threw his back out working for the "man."

Timmy will die soon.

Help Timmy because he won't help himself and he doesn't believe it is his fault. He thinks it is yours and you should pay for it.

By giving to The Timmy Fund you will help Timmy's family and their lawyer profit when he is gone.

The Timmy Fund
Helping the irresponsible die fat, lazy and bitter, but with a little change in their pocket.

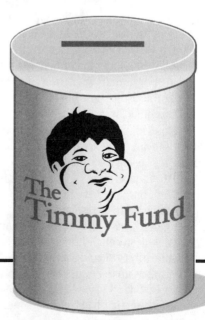

Have Stones, Will Travel

Mr. Jones was a 52-year-old white male who presented for an initial evaluation of flank pain. He seemed to be a pleasant, engaging, and intelligent man in appearance. He stated that he had a long history of nephrolithiasis (kidney stones) and he had seen several urologists in the past for these kidney problems. He reported that he recently had an ultrasound done by his last urologist that showed a stone in the uretero-pelvic junction. It was so thoughtful of him to carry this study with him to my office.

THOSE DARN NARC SEEKERS

It turns out that Mr. Jones was a Vietnam veteran having served with the infantry and did two tours of duty earning a purple heart and a bronze star for heroism. Having served in the army myself, as well as the infantry, I felt a connection with this pleasant man and admired his sense of duty and patriotism. We discussed the rest of his past medical history and I wrote him a prescription for Percocet for his pain. He told me that this medication was the only one that worked for him in the past. I subsequently set him up for a spiral CT scan of his urinary tract, as well as a trip to a local urologist for possible lithotripsy, as his stone was quite large.

Mr. Jones quickly spoke up and stated that he would not see any of the local urologists due to "interpersonal" conflicts with all three doctors. My ears went up as more red flags were flying right and left, but I did have in my hands a documented stone on an ultrasound. By this time his urinalysis came back with pinkish color and many RBCs (red blood cells). I referred him to a specialist in a nearby town and set him up with me for follow-up to discuss his progress. Later that day, I placed a call to one of the urologists that had "interpersonal"

problems with Mr. Jones. It turns out that Mr. Jones did in fact have a history of drug-seeking behavior and this urologist would no longer see him due to escalating usage and suspicious behavior.

Several days later, Mr. Jones called me for a refill on his Percocet. I had given him forty tablets, which should have lasted one or two weeks. When he came in, I recommended alternative medication, which he quickly blocked due to sensitivities to Toradol, Ultram, Ibuprofen, etc. He complained of escalating pain that ran along his flank down to the testicle on the same side as his stone showed on ultrasound. Repeat urinalysis did again show blood in the urine. Reluctantly, I gave him a second prescription for forty Percocet with no refills.

Several days later I got a call from my receptionist that Mr. Jones was in the waiting room with his Percocet bottle in his hand. It contained a milky white solution with pill fragments. Wouldn't you know it, his wife washed his pants containing the bottle of Percocet and now he needs a refill.

I put Mr. Jones in a room and read him the riot act. There would be no more narcotics of any sort prescribed to him. Mr. Jones became irate and he threatened bodily harm to me and my staff. He also threatened legal action and vowed to fight back against doctors who do not treat patients who have real pain. His swan song was so inspirational that I have a tear in my eye as I write this.

Several weeks later I received a phone call from the urologist to whom I had referred him. It seems good old Mr. Jones had used this same ultrasound, as well as some blood in the urine for good measure, to gain access to more Percocet from this seasoned urologist. I called Dr. Y to express my concern and to compare notes.

After realizing that he had been conned, he agreed that Mr. Jones would not receive any further narcotics from him.

Several months had gone by and I forgot about my sweet friend. It seems that Mr. Jones had disappeared off of the radar screen until one day my secretary buzzed me.

"Doctor, an Agent White of the Drug Enforcement Agency is on the phone and would like to talk to you."

After calming down enough to release my anal sphincter muscle, I got on the phone. The topic indeed was Mr. Jones and Agent White wanted to set up a meeting for the next day.

The agent informed me that Mr. Jones was a professional. He had hit twenty-six doctors in three states with his story and ultrasound. *He was obtaining Percocet at an average rate of 700 tablets per month!*

Mr. Jones was obviously not consuming this amount, so we assume he was selling these on the black market.

I felt like a fool.

The agent informed me that my prescribing habits were not unusual and that most doctors are compassionate and willing to give the patient the benefit of the doubt *(under his breath I am sure he really was calling me a dumbass).* Agent White informed me that Mr. Jones was uncovered due to the fact he used his own Medicaid numbers to obtain the prescriptions. Another example of our hard-earned tax dollars at work. Mr. Jones was going to jail for Medicaid fraud. I was going back to work.

Trust is an important part of the doctor-patient relationship. This guy must have pricked his finger in the bathroom to put blood in his urine. He traveled with his ultrasound like some would travel with their nitroglycerin because "you never know when you are going to need it."

I am sorry I trusted Mr. Jones, but you can't be distrustful of all patients.

Do you think he really earned a purple heart or bronze star for heroism?

Do you think monkeys are going to fly out of my ass? ✛

TOP TEN
Ways a Drug Rep Pisses Off a Physician

10 Reminiscent of *The Godfather*, he gives the doctor a trinket worth all of three cents and subsequently believes the doctor owes him a favor to be repaid some day.

9 She dresses up inappropriately, because in reality she is almost a model, and talks to the physician in a seductive manner *(actually we like that one).*

8 He places tons of useless paraphernalia and *"pseudo"* studies on the physician's desk and hopes the doctor doesn't catch him.

7 She tries to sit the physician down and teach him as if she were a professor putting the doctor through medical school again.

6 He begs the doctor to sit and listen to some ridiculous video or audio conference so she may receive a gift three months later *(which is actually a book written by their company).*

5 She uses hard-sell tactics that are so forceful it can be likened to kidnapping the doctor, throwing him into a van and deprogramming him as in some cult member rescue.

4 He dances and prances around the hallway and nearby the patients' rooms hoping the physician will get excited when she sees him when in actuality the doctor really wants to just jab his eye out with his company insignia pen.

3 She leaves propaganda in the waiting room that is so biased it may as well say, *"I lost 30 pounds in a week. Call me and ask me how."*

2 He out and out lies about his competitor's product and then denies he said it when questioned by the physician on the next visit. Three months later he changes companies and starts bad-mouthing his first company and product.

1 She moves her competitor's products around on the drug shelf like it is a side-street shell game, thinking the physician won't be able to find the other drug and therefore will pick hers. ✛

X-Ray Files

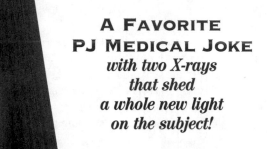

A FAVORITE PJ MEDICAL JOKE
with two X-rays that shed a whole new light on the subject!

A man went into the proctologist's office for his first exam. The doctor told him to have a seat in the examination room and that she would be with him in just a few minutes. When the man sat down and began observing the tools, he noticed there were items on a stand next to the doctor's desk:

a tube of K-Y jelly, a rubber glove, and a beer.

When the doctor finally came in, the man said, *"Look Doc, I'm a little confused. This is my first exam and I know what the K-Y is for, and I know what the glove is for, but can you tell me what the BEER is for?"*

At that, the doctor became noticeably outraged and stormed over to the door. The doc flung the door open and yelled to her nurse . . .

"Dammit, Helen! I said A BUTT LIGHT."

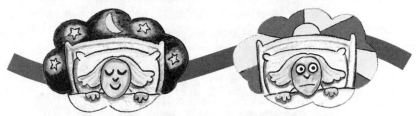
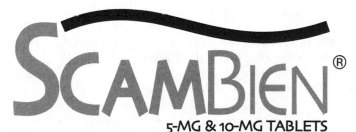

Yellow Bill

This Darn Narc Seeker is an interesting gentleman from the South. Yellow Bill was a 23-year-old male with lower back pain. Before coming to see me, he was treated for several years by an alleged pain specialist whose therapeutic plan consisted of weekly injections of undisclosed substances and a liberal hand with the prescription pad. At the time of referral he was on Norco, clonazepam and diazepam, among other things.

His physical examination was remarkable for bright yellow pointy hair (hence his nickname) and several decorative foreign body insertions. I tried not to be judgmental; after all, during the 70s I sported a rather Messianic appearance, the main purpose of which, looking back, was to:
(1) Get babes and
(2) Piss off old people.

I decided Bill was just a regular garden-variety Gen-X'er, or is it Gen-Y? At any rate, it was one of those chromosomes. I am pushing 50, but I'm not some old fogy. Well, I am, and I think Bill O'Reilly is God incarnate, but I'm not going to let these young pissants know that their stupid hair and body mutilations get to me. I gave Yellow Bill the benefit of the doubt, having somehow forgotten the prodigious consumption of mind-altering substances that went with my rebellious appearance 30 years ago, mostly in the pursuit of #1 (vide supra).

Yellow Bill successfully switched from Norco to a Duragesic-25 patch, which I took as a favorable sign, since Norco is much more fun. He also underwent several invasive procedures for his pain, including successful prognostic lumbar medial branch blocks, followed by good pain reduction with lumbar facet injections.

THOSE DARN NARC SEEKERS

He then developed radicular pain, which clinically and on EMG looked like L5 radiculopathy (spinal injury). We did selective L5 blocks with good relief. Bill seemed like a legitimate pain patient. With his pain under good control he was referred to physical therapy for reconditioning. I continued his Duragesic-25 patch and Zanaflex pending his physical therapy. I felt good. This is how pain management should be. I had renewed faith in my fellow (alleged) man.

After 23 years in medicine you'd think I'd learn. Three months after that visit, the pharmacy called to check on the dosage of three scripts my "office" had called in: seventy-five Vicodin, seventy-five diazepam with one refill, and forty-five phenobarbital with one refill. The alert pharmacist called because the phenobarbital was for 50 mg and they don't make a 50 mg pill. He wanted to know if we could substitute two 30 mg pills or three 15 mg pills. Talk about picking up on subtle discrepancies. This guy was a wiz with math.

Who called that in? Well, it was very busy at the pharmacy so they didn't write down a name. We informed the pharmacist that we do not call in scripts for controlled substances, and we certainly didn't call in that mess. It was suggested that perhaps a consultation from the local constabulary was in order.

When Yellow Bill showed up to pick up his prescription, the cops were there waiting with shiny new bracelets to go with his earrings. The police can be your best friends sometimes. I think Yellow Bill will be very popular in prison and have a lot of dates. For me, I can go back to being judgmental. ✚

THE
EXPERIENCED
DOCTOR

INTRODUCTION

"Dr. Farrago, your next patient is in the room."
"Great, what's the story?"
"Well, she is new to the practice. She just needs a referral to a neurologist. She said she goes to a methadone clinic because she used to be addicted to Vicoden."
"Oh."

Even though I was in a great mood, I was still a little leery about that last statement. But the fact that she fessed up to her narcotic addiction to my nurse did put me at ease. **Honesty from my patients is very important for the relationship.** I figured I would just go into the room with an open mind and lay down some simple ground rules if she wanted any pain medication from me.

As I walked into the room I saw the patient sitting comfortably in the chair. She was relaxed and in her mid-forties. She had appropriate attire on and was smiling. I looked at her, said hello and sat down. She looked somewhat familiar but, when I glanced at her name on the chart, I definitely didn't recognize it.

"What can I do for you today?" I asked.
"I just need to get a primary care doctor and a referral to a neurologist."
Simple enough. I shook my head and was about to speak. As I opened my mouth, it hit me. That voice! That face! I took a second and responded to her in a very calm but direct manner.
"Ma'am, I can't be your doctor. You have to go somewhere else for your care."
"But why!" she protested.
"Because the last time you were here you tried to choke me."

By the time you read this book I will have been practicing primary care medicine for more than a decade, but I am still in that transition period between being a new doctor and a fully experienced doctor. I think my reaction in the story above, which is entirely true, shows that I'm on my way. As a medical student, resident or new doctor, I might have called the police, yelled at the patient, screamed at my staff for letting her sneak back in, or left the office in a pissed-off mood. **As I get older, I realize that we can choose our reactions.** In this scenario, I chose to laugh about it and use it as a teaching tool. From what I've observed, this is what experienced doctors do.

When I first saw this patient, about two years earlier, she was drunk or hopped up on drugs when I declined to give her any medication. She became obnoxious and verbally abusive before lunging at me in an attempt to choke me as I escorted her from my office. The lisp in her speech tipped me off as I found myself again escorting her out into the hallway.

"Why did I try to choke you?" she asked.
"I actually don't know."
"Well, you must have done something to deserve it."

Physicians are humans and they go through all the emotions that anyone else does. What separates us from other professions is that we see into the most private and darkest parts of our patients' souls. Unfortunately, what we find there, along with years of torture at the hands of the medical axis of evil *(HMOs, pharmaceutical companies and medical malpractice insurers)*, may weigh heavily on our shoulders and drive some of us to burnout. **After years and years in practice, many physicians start to go off the deep end.**

124

There are those doctors who no longer smile. There are those doctors who no longer laugh. There are those that are socially withdrawn and don't talk much anymore to their colleagues. Many consider retirement about as often as they have dinner. Many are bitter toward the system and even their patients. They neglect to keep up with the advances of medicine. They have difficulty handling the new technological advances because they rebel against progress. Some become depressed. Marriages get shaky. Some remarry. Others become lonely. Many physicians put in impossible hours because being a doctor is all they know – they define themselves by their job and their self-worth is measured by how many hours they put in on the job. As their lives and their families fall apart, this sometimes leads them to question their choice of profession. I have seen doctors whose own health has suffered because they care for everyone but themselves. **This type of experienced doctor is the pessimist.** Their glass is always half-empty; in fact, they're usually pretty sure that someone stole their glass.

Luckily, there is another type of experienced doctor. They are the optimists. *These doctors continue on like a well-oiled machine. They know their patients and their idiosyncrasies and more importantly, they know their own. They are aware of what lines they can cross when they joke with patients because they have built solid relationships with them over the years. The minor stressors of the job roll off their backs. They are both efficient and effective on the job. They still care about medicine, but they also have a healthy outlook on life and have other interests outside the profession. They are financially secure and, unlike the burned-out physician, they are not working to support their own monetary indiscretions. They actually don't need to work anymore but continue because they enjoy it. They know that the job isn't perfect, but see it for what it is. These wise old owls have found peace.*

To these physicians, the glass is neither half-full nor half-empty. Their success and survival is based on the ability to experience the good and the bad equally without letting the worst parts get to them. Their glass is not lost but in fact created in a manner of their liking. They have molded it and it lasts forever.

This last section has lots of stories that will give you an idea of what it is like to be a physician for many years. Though many different specialties are represented, I can assure you that **all the stories are from optimists.** They are the doctors who will make you laugh and they are the ones I aspire to be like. **Humor is their best weapon to survive, and this is the common thread tying these stories together.** Perspective equals longevity when defining a long career in medicine. After decades in this arduous profession, these doctors truly tell the tales that show how they not only endured in their career choice but actually flourished in it. Some may do this with a joke, while the rest of us just try not to get choked.

✚

The Pareto Principle is in full effect in the practice of primary care medicine. You know the rule where you are more productive by concentrating on the most prioritized issues.

20% of your work is more important than the **80%** of the other stuff.

I think we can apply that in another way on our job. **20%** of our patients take up more than **80%** of our time. The problem is that those **20%** are the neediest.

They are not necessarily bad people, but they do need a lot of attention. What makes this worse, however, is the fact that these patients are the most annoying and give you the least satisfaction on the job. These are the same patients that complain the most, have the most admissions, and are the least happy with your care.

In fact, you have to almost neglect the other **80%** in order to handle these **20%**.

This happens to all of us without exception.

PJ EXPLAINS
THE 80/20 RULE OF MEDICINE

Some rules are hard to break.

Let's add more to the mix. These are the patients that give you the most gastritis on the job. They are your narcotic seekers, chronic complainers, somatosizers, and are the least appreciative of your help. They are the first to fire you. They are the first to complain when you don't give them all the attention or are late to their appointments.

It does not matter how successful you were in the past either.

"Oh, Doctor, you were so great today spending all that time with me."

The one time you had to concentrate on another emergency and had to speed up their appointment or even worse, didn't return their call about the boil situated on the crest of their gluteal cleft, you get . . .

"Doctor X never gives me enough time. I deserve more. Send me my records!"

Sure, they may let one "episode" where you neglected them slide, but it will haunt you later. These patients keep a scorecard and have no statute of limitations. You can never win because you were set up to lose from the get-go. These patients have the worst disease that is caused by their own destructive behaviors or are the ones that have the fewest "real" symptoms. They are also the ones who will doctor shop and leave you at any time for someone who really "cares" (and subsequently leave that doctor in one year's time).

80% of the time they have nothing you can really treat, but **20%** of the time they may have something that needs real medical help.

For that reason, you are medically liable if you ignore that headache that is actually a malignant tumor. It is because of this you never give up on them because of doctor guilt and therefore, you keep trying.

The **80%** of patients you have that are basically healthy, but need help occasionally, get the least of your attention because they are relatively easy. They are hardworking and from solid families and are a breath of fresh air when you walk into the exam room. These are the ones that almost make you feel weird because they are so normal. You walk out of the room energized and wish you could have stayed longer, but unfortunately you had to go see Mr. Gibbons with his backache of thirty years, or Mrs. Myers with chronic dizziness.

How does one rectify this situation?

One way not to fix it is to hire a midlevel provider. Not that there is anything wrong with them. They definitely fill a niche in a busy practice. Unfortunately, many physicians use them as a way to clear out the easier cases or "low-lying fruit." Sure you may think that they handle your extra volume, but they are actually getting to see the **80%** of your practice that makes the job enjoyable. This again leaves the needy **20%** with you!

A slow and insidious death for most practitioners occurs at that point. The hourglass turns over until one day all the sand is out and you're selling crafts at a mall boutique because you needed a change.

We at *Placebo Journal* recommend that you embrace your midlevel practitioners with open arms by setting them up with your "chronics." They couldn't do worse than you anyway. Let them taste this aspect of our job in all its glory. You can then sit back with your **80%** of "normals" and from time to time huddle and reflect with your midlevels on how they are doing. When you are done laughing, pat them on the back and give them a little reassurance. Welcome them into the "club" and state "welcome to real medicine." When they quit, we would then recommend you get cardboard cutouts of doctors *(see offer below)* with real empathic facial gestures to spend all the time in the world with your needy **20%**.

Your friend, PJ ✚

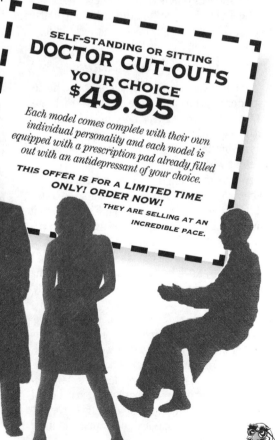

DOCTOR, I CAN'T KEEP IT UP MUCH LONGER...

Patients should take a more active role in their health . . .

Everyone knows the type, the patient who has no idea what medicine they are on or what they take that "little blue pill" for. It just seems odd to our anal retentive minds that they can be so clueless! So, when you meet a patient like Mr. X *(no, that isn't his real name)*, it makes you feel good that there are indeed normal patients out there. I am an anesthesiologist practicing in a mid-sized New England hospital and take pride in what I do and how I interact with my patients.

I introduced myself to Mr. X and explained the plan for general anesthesia and reviewed his chart. I had him sign his consent form and ordered the standard pre-op meds. Mr. X was a very nice elderly gentleman with end-stage lung disease and was totally ventilator dependent. Don't get me wrong, his limiting medical condition didn't seem to suppress his enthusiasm for life at all.

He was an inspiration.

He had a very compact, quiet, portable home ventilator that he could close off at his trach site and force air through his larynx and talk quite well. Preoperatively he could manage his vent himself, but I asked him to go over the ventilator's functions with me as most likely he would be somewhat sedated in the recovery room and unable to operate it. It was quite simple to use and it would be easy for me to put him back on it upon leaving the operating room. After answering a few other minor questions, I went back to sit down in the anesthesia office as my chart work was ready, my anesthesia circuit and machine had been turned over and all of my drugs were ready for this next case.

While drinking my morning juice and talking with some department members in the office, the front OR desk let me know they were calling for the patient to come over to the holding area. I said, "Thank you for letting me know." A few minutes later I was informed that he had arrived but they would not be moving him directly to the OR because the surgical team wasn't quite ready.

Again I thanked them for the information and asked them to let me know when he was going to the OR as I was all ready.

Five or ten minutes had gone by and again the front desk reminded me that he was in the holding area. It is nice that they are so attentive. Once again I thanked them for the information and reminded them that all they had to do was let me know when they were actually moving him into the OR. I thought their constant prompting was now getting a little odd, but I dismissed it and went back to my conversation.

Another five or ten minutes went by and the front desk nurse manager came to the anesthesia office door again. This time she looked a little flustered and reported that,

"The patient is starting to get tired."

I said, *"Excuse me, he's tired?"* Perplexed, I looked at my partners and reluctantly got up to see what the so-called troublesome problem was. Upon arriving to the holding area I saw immediately in front of the OR desk what the problem was. There was Mr. X, no home ventilator in sight, looking up at me with his kind eyes and **SQUEEZING HIS OWN AMBU BAG!**

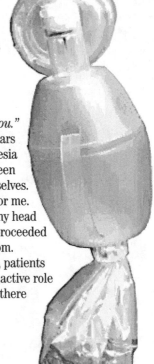

Realizing he had been doing this for some time now, I happily took over bagging for him. He looked up and mouthed, *"Thank you."*

In seven plus years of providing anesthesia I have never, ever seen a patient bag themselves. That was a record for me. With that, I shook my head with disbelief and proceeded to the operating room.

As I said before, patients should take a more active role in their health, but there are some limits. ✚

BE CAREFUL!

Several years ago I was putting an 80-year-old lady on warafin anticoagulation. She was about to go home from the hospital and I was giving her my usual spiel about avoiding alcohol, calling me before she took any new drug, and trying to keep a consistent diet.

I had just eaten lunch in the doctors' dining room and listened to some pediatricians talking about a baby born with birth defects typical of warfarin – another hazard with the drug that I may have known but forgotten because most of my patients can't remember back as far as their last period. At the end of my spiel, I thought I'd be cute and told the old lady, *"Oh, and don't get pregnant."*

She looked me straight in the eye, and said, ***"I'll be REAL careful!"*** ✚

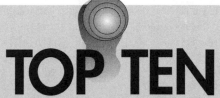

TOP TEN
Things Your Mother Always Told You to Do That You Wish Patients Listened To

10 Always wear clean underwear.

9 Brush your teeth twice a day.

8 Don't smoke.

7 Take regular showers or baths.

6 Don't pick at it!

5 Wipe good!

4 Always wash your hands after using the bathroom.

3 Don't play with sharp objects.

2 Cover your mouth when you cough.

1 Don't touch that or you'll go blind.

PHYSICIAN, HEEL THYSELF

A father recently came in with his son begging for the child to receive antibiotics. The kid looked healthier than me. I was at a point in my day that I could probably be persuaded into prescribing anything. As I sat listening to the father go on and on with a totally nebulous story, my mind began to wander. Thoughts in my head included *"What is that noise in the hallway?"* and *"Gee, I'm getting fat."* What brought me out of my coma were the father's implied demands for treatment. *"In my opinion, he has walking pneumonia."* Personally, I can't stand it when a patient thinks they have the real diagnosis and is just coming in to see me as a formality; especially when that diagnosis is totally made up.

What the hell is walking pneumonia anyway? Is that an old Indian term, kind of like Chief Running Stream? Welcome to our office Chief Walking Pneumonia.

The bottom line was that the kid had clear lungs, clean ears, and a negative rapid strep test (I do this sometimes as a way to convince the patient that it's viral).

As the father continued with his diatribe it suddenly hit me that it was his wife who had called my employers about a month earlier complaining about her visit. She had felt rushed *(even though we squeezed her in on a busy day as an acute)* and felt that I didn't do much for her *(she had a cold)*. We tried to call her back but she never responded. So here I am with this lady's kid who has a little virus *(emphasis on little)* and I just knew I was being tested to see if I would come through with the goods *(the goods being a nice little Z-Pak)*. As the father pushed, I began to dig in my heels. *I actually don't wear heels as I am a man, but for the purpose of this story please picture that I have 10-inch heels dug deep into the ground. Picture them being mauve while you're at it (but that's another story).*

He continued with his "evidence" stating that a virus wouldn't last two or three weeks *(it would)* and that Chief Walking Pneumonia needed something to cure him. Every time I would state a reason why not to treat with antibiotics he would counter with a reason to use antibiotics.

 For example, I would say that his lungs are clear and he would say that CWP (Chief Walking Pneumonia) has a bad cough. I would say that it doesn't seem that bad and he would say you should have heard him an hour ago. I would say that there is no fever and he would say that last night CWP was very warm. I would say that his ears and throat are normal and he would say that it gets worse at the end of the day. We volleyed back and forth for five minutes, but I wasn't giving in. Finally, I closed the interview with the obligatory advice to call us if things got worse but that it still might take a while to finally clear – as it was a virus.

The father of CWP wasn't happy and actually, neither was I. I don't really want to fight with patients *(I can do that with my family)*. I really try to bust my butt to get patients in that are sick. That, unfortunately, isn't enough for some. I remember my former attendings stating that good communication and education about viruses would help this type of problem. *Bullsh$t!* I could have tutored this guy for an hour and it wouldn't have mattered. He wanted those antibiotics.

After work my partners and I were debriefing, as we often do. I was retelling this story to one of my partners and made a point of stating how good our office is in getting people in the same day they call *(of course we don't do anything once we see them)*. He immediately chimed in that we use our "fund of knowledge" to reassure patients and that is what CWP's father was paying for. Basically what he was saying is that many times all we do is bless our patients. I thought to myself, if that is true then what I really need to do is bring my white jacket into the tailor's office and have flowing robes added to it. When I walk into the room with the patient I can do my exam and then dim the lights for special effects. With a loud voice and a British accent I can say, *"I, Sir Douglas Farrago MD, declare you . . . WELL!"* and then leave the room. Or I could just give the freakin' antibiotics. ✚

ADDENDUM: *Later on that week the mother needed her other son seen. As usual, we put the kid in and my nurse told her up front on the phone that it would have to be quick because we were going to be swamped. She showed up later that day with flowers for each staff member and myself. Her kid had conjunctivitis and got antibiotics. I blessed him and off they went. Sometimes it's not a virus.*

HIHOWAAHYA?

BOWEL OBSESSION

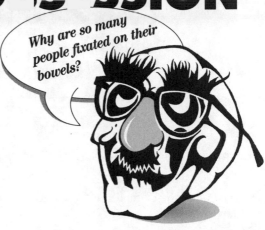

Why are so many people fixated on their bowels?

I have had patients in my time that are so obsessed with their bowels that they have decided the world revolves around their stool. I remember one patient had to explain every little cramp she had in her abdomen. And the gas! *Terrible*. The stool was just not the right color brown for her and it seems size does matter. After dealing with her constipation on a regular basis, I finally came to the realization that maybe I was never going to help her. She was always going to have something to complain about. The stools were too loose, too hard, too thin or not long enough. Like Goldilocks, except it was never just right.

I know this whole topic seems immature for a physician to talk about, but the problem is that it is all too common. Some doctors label these patients with a diagnosis of "Irritable Bowel Syndrome." I am not a big believer in this term, as there seems to be a huge supratentorial component. Even the name "Irritable Bowel" is ridiculous. If you want to have some fun, try this. Talk as if you were a pirate and repeat after me, *"You don't want to mess with him, matey, he's got eerrrtibill bowwwelllll."* Or pretend you are in a bar fight and state to the biker that is in your face, *"Back off buddy, I've got irritable bowel."*

The bottom line is that you cannot fix the unfixable. Try giving them laxatives, bulk formers, and antispasmodics. Try changing their diet, as more fiber should help. Try something for stress, an SSRI or counseling. Try, try, and try. The truth is that every conversation will begin the same way and end the same way. Their bowel movements are never perfect. It is as if they are looking for the perfect stool much as a surfer looks for the perfect wave. *Man, that was a Tsunami turd!*

Now we all have those times that good bowel movement makes your day. You feel light and airy and that post-parasympathetic high feels great. There is nothing wrong with that. These people, however, are on a quest for Nirvana and looking for it via their rectum.

STOOL SAMPLES

WRONG COLOR

TOO THIN

TOO LOOSE

TOO HARD

TOO SHORT

TSUNAMI TURD

You have choices. You could always send them to a gastroenterologist, but that would be dumping (no pun intended). I am sure specialists don't want to deal with these patients either. Maybe an alternative practitioner would work? *"How about some Eye of Newt, Mrs. Jones?"* It really doesn't matter. Anywhere you send them will only be temporary because, like a boomerang, they return.

So how do we deprogram these patients who are being brainwashed by their bowels?

I recommend that physicians learn the art of distraction. Just like a good magician, never have them focus on that which they want. When they talk constipation, you talk about their eyes. When they mention gas, you go on a soliloquy about their dry skin. When they mention stool caliber, you mention joint laxity. You can get so good at this that you will have five things to talk to them about before they can even hit you about their bowels. Like a role reversal, you now have the "list" and you go into each visit on the offensive. This stuff works. Then again, if it doesn't, there is always the gastroenterologist.

Your friend, PJ ✚

TOP TEN

Ways to Get "Hunkered Down" Patients Out of the Hospital

10 Cut off all power to the room and pump in loud rock music *(sort of like we did with General Noriega)*.

9 Three letters – ECT (electroconvulsive therapy, or shock to the brain).

8 Low calorie, soft mechanical, low salt, low fat, low sugar, low taste, and puréed diet.

7 Send in a new medical student every hour on the hour to ask for a full review of systems and to perform a full complete physical exam *(including checking Cranial Nerve I with coffee grinds)*.

6 Hourly enemas.

5 Admit your favorite patient with sleep apnea or with dementia *(that tends to sundown a bit)* to the bed next to them.

4 If patient is a female – only have ESPN on the tube; if patient is a male – only have Lifetime on the tube.

3 Have interns master the skill of getting arterial blood gasses on this patient.

2 Have maintenance come in and install a "dripping" faucet.

1 Have nurse attempt to insert largest size urethral catheter he or she can find *(easily found at a nearby large animal veterinarian's office)*.

Over 30 years ago, I started my general practice in a small southern town of around 2,000 people. My first attempt began while moonlighting in a small, rented two-bedroom house. A radiological resident and I made the small office with no air conditioner and a gas space heater into our place of business. We furnished it with cheap plastic chairs and indoor-outdoor carpet from Sears. *We were styling.* Office visits were $7. Since malpractice insurance was only $130 a year, we weren't in bad shape.

One of our first patients was a white middle-class lady who brought her child in with a cold. What was nice was the fact that she really was there to support the venture of the two "new doctors" since the community hadn't had a physician in several years. Unfortunately, she became very uncomfortable with the dumpy surroundings and the odor from the poorly ventilated space heater. She never returned.

The next patient was an elderly black man who brought in his own special smell, that being the wood smoke with which he heated his own home. With complete sincerity, and even a sense of awe, he volunteered, *"I really likes your house."*

My partner, the radiological resident, had his own issues. He bought a well-used portable X-ray machine from a tech at the nearby army post. The price included the tank for hand development. It took about 20 minutes to get "wet readings." We jimmy-rigged the back porch to block the light out. This made it into a Plywood X-Ray Suite. The initial films took more than ten minutes to get a poor image at best. It took awhile for my partner to realize that he shouldn't leave the paper on the individually wrapped films. Once he started taking the paper off, the picture quality was actually pretty good and we were up and going.

Our first chance to get the Plywood X-Ray Suite some action came days later when a small older lady needed some chest images. Our film cassettes were black with an aluminum colored band around them. She stood in front of the cassette as instructed and while we were taking the film, she commented, *"Sho is dark out tonight."* I nodded but really wasn't paying much attention until she jumped back, covered herself and blurted out *"They took the window down!"* when my employee removed the cassette that was in front of her.

Life was different then. And more simple. Rufus epitomized this "simpleness." He began to appear at our clinic on a regular basis. His life was chaotic but happy. He spent his disability checks on lottery tickets. He usually lived in someone's barn or shed and was fed by the kindness of others. For 20 years he had insulin-dependent diabetes and nary a clue how to adjust his medicine or diet. He walked 20 miles most days and we would see him all over the county walking alongside the road. The only time he would get into trouble and need an admission to the hospital was when he was able to acquire an old broken-down car. This came as a result of some do-gooder convincing him to get a driver's license (which he did). How he passed the test without being able to read or write was beyond me. Unfortunately, the walking had prevented him from going into diabetic ketoacidosis so when he drove his car he got sicker. The beauty about Rufus was his carefree style. It would not be uncommon to overhear him propose to the local bank manager knowing well and good she was already married with children. The one thing, however, that I always envied about Rufus was his watch. It had no hands (and wasn't digital). Time stood still for this man – not unlike how time stands still for my old memories.

✛

NEW DOC VS.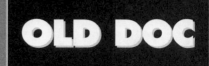

There is more here than meets the eye.	There is less here than meets the eye.
I need to do an extensive review of symptoms.	A review of systems can only get me into trouble.
Sure she has some narcotic seeking behavior but I need to trust my patients.	Get the hell out of my office.
I wish I could spend more time with my patients to really get inside their heads.	I wish I could spend less time with my patients because I can't get them out of my head.
My staff needs constant positive feedback and I will do this by catching them doing something right.	My staff and I have been together so long that if they weren't pulling their weight I would have thrown them out years ago.
These drug reps really have some good information to offer me.	Get these damn drug reps out of the office or I'll . . . a free concert ticket? OK, what drug do you have?
This case is so complicated that I need to call the specialist to ask his advice.	This case is so ridiculous that I need to call the specialist to see if he needs a laugh.
Do you have anything else I can help you with ma'am?	Next!
Bring them right in; I can handle that right here in the office.	Tell them to suck it up or else go to the freakin' ER.
What your teenager needs is some good TLC.	What your teenager needs is a good beating.
This dictation for a complete physical will take about 30 minutes. Thank goodness I can use a template on my electronic medical records program.	Healthy. Return in a year.
I hope Medicare pays the full amount.	Cash only.
I really need to cut my hours to spend more time with my family.	I am working my ass off so my family can spend the money without me.

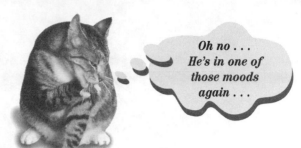

Oh no . . . He's in one of those moods again . . .

Here Kitty, Kitty...

Our small rural hospital does not have house physicians or residents, so the handful of general internists on staff rotate "Medical Call" and "ICU Call" for unassigned patients. One evening, I was called to the ER to admit a man after an unsuccessful suicide attempt. The man was gay, about 60, and lived alone except for an undetermined number of cats. He was a diabetic with some heart disease, and was dating a doctor who did not have privileges at our hospital (naturally!).

He was evidently upset with his life and current boyfriend, and so decided to end it all (after a few too many drinks). He had heard that a person could die from too much insulin, but he wasn't sure how much was needed, so first, he injected one of his cats with about 50 units of regular. The cat began seizing sometime afterward, and died, but he really didn't like the way that looked, so he decided to try another method.

He went to the garage, taking another cat with him, I guess thinking of the canary in a mine idea. He and the cat sat in the car with the engine running, and as he got sleepier, the cat became frantic, keeping him from relaxing adequately. He then started to get nauseated, so he shut off the car, and he and the cat went back into the house.

Then he decided to slit his wrists, but after a few ineffectual superficial cuts (it hurt!), he tried stabbing himself in the chest, resulting in another superficial wound, which also hurt (but at least no cats died this time).

He then thought about the electrical appliance in the bathtub idea, and so filled the tub, brought the toaster into the bathroom, making sure he had an adequate extension cord, got in, and plonked in the toaster. The circuit breaker tripped, and that was it.

At that point, he evidently decided that it was not a good day to die, and so he came to the ER, had his wounds stitched and bandaged, and I admitted him to the ICU, thinking that this was probably the strangest, most pathetic story of suicide I had ever heard.

The next day, on early rounds, he was sitting up in his bed eating breakfast, and I told him that we would arrange for a psychiatrist to see him as he was no longer in any medical danger. I left the room to make some notes in his chart when he called me back with a loud *"Hey, Doc."*

As I stepped in, he pointed to the bacon and eggs he was eating from the regular diet I had inadvertently ordered, and said: *"Hey Doc, I'm supposed to be on a low fat diet! Are you trying to kill me?"* ✚

135

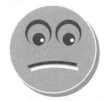 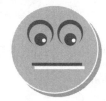
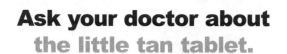

PJ PHARMACEUTICALS
asks the question,
"Who really is that happy anyway?"

PJ PHARMACEUTICALS   1000 mg

:|Indifferex:)©

Because even your doctor
doesn't care that much.

Warning: What you should know about
the safety of Indifferex©

May cause gas, a purplish color tinge to your testicles
(if you have them) and death.
Indifferex© really is a farce. If you choose to believe this
you are a complete idiot.

PJ PHARMACEUTICALS   1000 mg

:|Indifferex:)©

The mediocre antidepressant

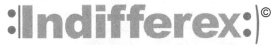

PJ PHARMACEUTICALS
©2003 PJ PHARMACEUTICALS Auburn, ME

PJ SAYS:
SUCK IT UP!

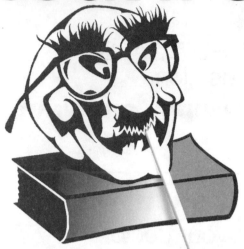

THE PAIN OF LIFE

In my day, there wasn't so much complaining. *Okay, maybe there was,but people at least kept quiet about it.* Nowadays everyone and their uncle has a problem that is in need of a treatment and they want it right away. It now seems that it is so acceptable to have a disease or syndrome that physicians are making new ones up just to make their patients happy . . . *or to shut them up.*

How all of a sudden depression becomes an epidemic is beyond me. Has the world changed that much? I think not. We just have more specialists. Every one of their recommendations states that this country's depression is undertreated. With every other patient on an SSRI already, how could that possibly be? If everyone including neonates had a 100 percent antidepressant use, I wonder whether these specialists would finally say that general practitioners are finally doing a good job. *I bet they would just find something else to bitch about.* Pretty soon HMOs will be checking the doctors' charts like they do for immunizations to see that all their patients are on something to make them happy.

Now pain specialists have gotten into the game. **They state that pain is the fifth vital sign.** I have no freakin' idea what the hell the other four are. They expect nurses to ask every patient about their pain and mark it in their chart. Pretty soon the nurses will be lying like they do about respiration rate. Respiration rate, there's one of the four other vital signs. Anyway, just like respiration rate, doctors will ignore it until lawyers start to sue. If it was up to lawyers and pain specialists every patient would be on narcotics until they were gorked out of their heads. Not too gorked or again the lawyers would sue. Do you see the constant theme here? Lawyers always sue.

What is wrong with just plain old sucking it up?

Not every patient needs antidepressants. They need to get their damn life together. They need to stop smoking and drinking. They need to start working, start eating better, start exercising, and start concentrating on the good things in life. No one was guaranteed happiness in the Constitution but instead "the pursuit of happiness." *Patients just need to get off their asses and pursue it.* Sure there are bad things that happen to them. There are bad things that happen to me (*I'm a skull*). **If there weren't bad things, no one actually would know what a good thing was because there would be nothing to compare it to.** Sure patients have some pain. *Are they doing anything about it?* I am not talking about metastatic cancer pain here. **I am talking about the pain of life.** How coincidental that the higher the stress in the life the higher the pain. *How many patients are just fat and out of shape?* When they don't move more than from the kitchen to the crapper then their bodies get more obese and their muscles just shrivel away. It's a vicious cycle and the only one that can fix it is the patient. Not the doctor. Not the antidepressant. Not the painkiller. **Only the patient – who has to suck it up!**

Okay, some people do have severe pain and severe depression but not 50 to 90 percent. *Please.*

Could it be that these same pain and depression specialists are just in pain about their career choice and now are depressed about what to do about it? *I have the same advice for them. Suck it up!* And leave the rest of us alone. ✚

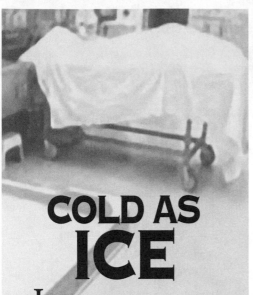

COLD AS
ICE

It was around three in the morning when the phone rang. It was the charge nurse from a nursing home. She told me she *"thought"* Mrs. Jones was dead. I asked what she meant by she *"thought"* the patient was dead. She said she just wasn't sure (*it says a lot about her training*).

After ascertaining that the patient was a DNR (do not resuscitate) and didn't appear to be in any distress, I told the nurse to leave Mrs. Jones where she was and call me in the morning if she hadn't moved.

Mrs. Jones didn't move, thus clinching the diagnosis of being dead. Shortly after this incident the nurse left the nursing profession. I was told she got a job on an assembly line. ✚

EDITOR'S NOTE - *Just another example why experience is everything.*

CREAMS DON'T WORK

Near the end of a hectic clinic day, the daughter of one of my regulars (a college sophomore) came in with a bad case of vaginitis. She'd tried one of those over-the-counter antifungal creams, but still had the itch and cottage-cheese discharge.

The story started when she had recently finished a course of Augmentin for an upper respiratory infection and had been started on oral contraceptives by the university health service. In other words, it was a set-up for moniliasis (yeast). The Chemstrip yielded a normal glucose. The subsequent speculum exam and wet mount/KOH confirmed moniliasis without any evidence of co-infection. We had the right diagnosis.

When I asked if she would like a prescription cream versus suppositories, she opted for the suppositories because *"the creams don't work!"* I wrote a prescription for Terazol suppositories, one at bedtime for three nights. The next morning, arriving before the rest of the staff and annoyed by the phone's recurrent and insistent ringing, I finally took the call. *Big mistake.* Our gal, after one night of therapy wanted something else. When I asked her why (worried about a potential adverse reaction) she informed me *"they're too damn hard to swallow!!"* Take home message: Never assume, always specify the route of administration. ✚

EDITOR'S NOTE:
What was her major?
Pre-Law?

THE DOCTOR'S

PATIENTS AND PUBLIC

The other day I came home after a miserable weekend on call where I covered ER and inpatient service at my local hospital. When I came home, my wife was writing something in a notebook that I found hysterical. After reading it, I proclaimed that this was definitely *Placebo Journal* material. It is something I wish I could publish in our newspaper. It goes like this . . .

1 I am not on call 24 hours a day, 7 days a week. Do not call my home to ask if I am on call either!

2 I have a personal life, and many times I do not give a rat's ass about your piddly problems.

3 DO NOT confront me in local or non-local establishments about you or your family's

  a. Abdominal pain
  b. Allergies
  c. Cough
  d. Colds, congestion
  e. Depression
  f. Anxiety
  g. Personal or marital problems
  h. Med refills
  i. Constipation
  j. Free consultations
  k. Weight loss/gain
  l. Diabetes
  m. Hypoglycemia (no such thing anyway)
  n. Blood pressure updates
  o. Pregnancy related problems
    p. Off the cuff Viagra prescriptions

  q. Nausea, vomiting
  r. STD
  s. Heartburn
  t. Mama in the nursing home
  u. Bleeding
  v. Strains, sprains, or pain
  w. Bipolar disorder
  x. Self-diagnosis you want me to validate
  y. Referrals
  z. Why you can't pay me
  aa. Why you still are coughing up a lung, but can't stop smoking
  bb. Drug problems
  cc. Rashes anywhere on your body.

4 I do not see hospital patients unless I am on freakin' call. If it is not my call night, I don't give a damn if you are the President's mom, DON'T EVEN ASK!!!

5 Repercussions for these infractions include:
  a. My wife can be a real bitch, and I will have her rail on you.
  b. You will receive a $50 per minute itemized billing sheet. And if you don't pay, refer to the above!

6 Do not bring any relatives with you to your office visit, and try to sneak in a free visit using the *"oh by the way . . ."* method. This is a very serious aggravation for me; it might set off my heretofore latent bipolar mood disorder. *(It's very popular to have it now, so I should jump on the bandwagon.)*

RULES

BE ADVISED

7 If you have an appointment with me, you are expected to arrive on time. NO EXCEPTIONS. "No-shows" are billed at double rate, payable in cash to my wife. If you are late to your appointment, you are SOL, and will still be billed. Again, payable in cash to my wife.

8 My phone rings 29 times a day, at least, and that is after hours. I have installed a state of the art feature that requires the caller to dial in his credit card number for $20 a minute. I hope this will significantly cut down on the calls from acquaintances and neighbors who think they have carte blanche access to free advice.

9 DO NOT come to my front door either!!! I have trained rottweillers, pit bulls, and brahma bulls. Also, there are armed booby traps, if you don't drown in my alligator-infested moat first.

10 Furthermore, do not complain to my office manager that my wife gave you a *"go to hell"* look last Saturday when you came to our table while we were having lunch with our three young boys, and decide to go into graphic detail about your vaginal bleeding (true story). You were VERY lucky that she only looked at you and did not subsequently beat the living hell out of you.

11 I have frequent memory lapses. So do not expect me to recall:

a. Who the hell you are.
b. Who your daddy is (I don't care).
c. Your every illness, medication, and dosage.

This is why we have a damn medical chart. I do not know what in the hell that little white pill you take every morning is. All pills are white, pink, blue, orange, and typically are round, or possibly square or triangular. Maybe you think I am a f#cking genie in a bottle? Oh, wait, maybe I am, and then I can grant your three wishes:

1. XANAX
2. SOMA
3. VICODIN

Here is a recent example that may help you:

For the first time in nearly four years, I called in sick with a fever of 104 degrees. Of course, by noon, I had already gotten several phone calls from you people with complaints in far lesser severity than what I was suffering. Believe it or not, I get sick too. But, I do not immediately report to the ER with my sore throat, or headache, especially at 4 a.m.!!

I look forward to providing medical care to you and yours. Our physician/patient relationship should be one of warmth and kindness, if the above-mentioned guidelines are strictly followed.

Respectfully,
Your Small Town Doctor
(as written by his wife) +

EDITOR'S NOTE: It could have been written by my wife as well.

141

Trader Jack was a worker's comp case with post-laminectomy syndrome, which is a polite term for failed back surgery that we use in order to not piss off the spine surgeons who refer these messes. He underwent the usual round of epidurals, nerve blocks, trials of co-analgesics, etc., without relief. I started him on chronic opiate therapy, and methadone seemed to work the best for him.

Eventually he wasn't satisfied with that and we had a few go-rounds about whether to increase his meds or try something more aggressive. He had a successful spinal cord stimulator trial, and that was followed by a permanent implant. Then he was pretty much on autopilot, using the stimulator, with methadone for breakthrough pain. *Or so I thought.*

One day I happened to be looking out the window into the parking lot when Jack pulled up . . . on his motorcycle. I asked him about how a guy with so much back pain could ride a Harley.

"Oh, riding my Harley makes my back feel good!" was the response.

This is a guy who is on the government teat with social security and disability.

I pulled out my trusty spinal cord stimulator programmer and interrogated his unit. On these models you can get a report of total use since initial activation.

THOSE DARN NARC SEEKERS

Trader Jack was using his stimulator one percent of the time. I asked him about this.

"I only use the stimulator when I'm at home," he explained.

"Jack," said I, *"even Dick Cheney, who is always running off to hide in 'undisclosed locations,' is home more than that. I think it's time to tinkle in this plastic cup."*

Well, Jack threw a fit. He refused to give a urine specimen, but he also refused to leave without a refill of his methadone. Finally I told him he could (1) leave, (2) give the sample, or (3) be escorted out by the police.

He gave a urine sample, which came back on our office testing kit as negative for methadone and positive for opiates and THC. I figured Trader Jack was swapping methadone for Vicodin and so I refused to give him a refill.

As with most sociopaths, he was very angry with me for catching him and he changed doctors.

When the new doc requested our records, the last office note was prominently displayed on the top of the pile.

I never heard from the "Trader" again. ✚

MY FAVORITE
MUNCHAUSEN

Ashlyn was 52 years old and suffering. For five years she had dealt with a vaginal discharge that would not go away. *Do you know how hard that must have been?* No one seemed to be able to cure her ills. Sure, her symptoms were complicated. Sure, the discharge was "different." But shouldn't Ashlyn be afforded the proper medical treatment to alleviate her complaints?

Here is the scoop. Ashlyn had a brown to black vaginal discharge. It supposedly didn't smell. It supposedly didn't itch. It did cause vaginal discomfort. Even worse, it stained all of Ashlyn's underwear which was not only embarrassing but quite costly.

Ashlyn's medical history was simple. She was married with four children.

She didn't drink, but she did smoke about 20 cigarettes a day. She had had an appendectomy, a D&C, a vaginal prolapse repair, a tubal ligation, and a hysterectomy. All pelvic exams were normal and vaginal swabs were negative. Her underwear did have an "unnatural black discoloration of the crotch area." *Hmmmm.*

Ashlyn also had some other history. Between 1981 and 1994, she had 65 specialist consultations including the likes of gynecology, urology, rheumatology, and cardiology. Extensive workups of the blood as well as radiological procedures never turned up anything. The 16 hospital admissions all were diagnoses-free as well. Oh yes, there were the 12

minor surgical procedures that turned up empty for pathology also.

One of the investigators got suspicious and decided to smell the underwear. *This, it seems, was in the interest in science.* We are not proponents of all physicians smelling the underwear of patients as this can be construed as, well, unprofessional. In this case, however, our heroes made an interesting finding.

The garment smelled like cigarette ash.

Off to the lab our heroes went (with the underwear) and the results soon came back. The toluene extract of the stain matched that of cigarette ash.

Our little Ashlyn seemed to have found a new way to put her cigarettes out. *Who needs ash trays when your vagina will do?* As they say in those cigarette commercials, *"You've come a long way, baby!"*

SOMETHING DOESN'T SMELL RIGHT

As weird as this may sound, Ashlyn denied the whole thing when confronted. To this day, the authors state she continues to see specialists for persisting urinary symptoms, rectal bleeding, etc. Unfortunately, none of those specialists were psychiatrists. The authors warn others of the financial burden that people like Ashlyn (Munchausens) put on the system. We agree and hope physicians out there get a little suspicious when someone asks for a nicotine inhaler to be used vaginally. ✚

Taken with liberties from European Journal of Obstetrics and Gynecology and Reproductive Biology *72 (1997) 105-106.*

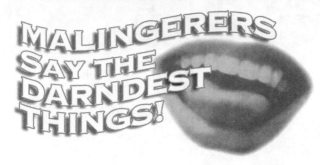

MALINGERERS SAY THE DARNDEST THINGS!

"HEAR TODAY, GONE TOMORROW"

I am an otolaryngologist in a medium-sized town. There are plenty of industrial jobs in the area. A 20-year-old male, whom we will call Mr. Blake, came to my office complaining of hearing loss in his right ear. He stated that it was due to a blow to the head that occurred at work. Off the bat he was setting this up to be a worker's compensation case.

On exam, his right tympanic membrane looked completely normal. An audiogram did show a slight sensorineural hearing loss, but the different parts of the exam just did not align properly. The audiologist was the first to be suspicious and made me aware.

When I reported the results to the patient, I used my usual strategy of telling him that the abnormalities of the test could be our fault. Maybe we didn't explain the instructions well or didn't motivate him to try hard enough. After putting him at ease, I invited him back to repeat the test on another day. In my experience, patients either never return (*because they were faking*) or return and get a totally normal exam (*because they were faking*).

Our friend returned for his second appointment. I gave his ears another look-see to make sure there wasn't any pathology I missed on the prior appointment (*there wasn't*). His canals were clean and his tympanic membranes were normal and mobile. Mr. Blake asked me again what had gone wrong with the first audiogram. I further explained that the different parts of the test just weren't consistent with each other. I directed him to my audiologist to repeat the exam once more.

After an hour and a half, I realized that he hadn't returned to my office. I called the audiologist to see what was going on. It seems Mr. Blake made it down the hallway, but not before stuffing a little piece of cotton in his ear. This was picked up by the audiologist who looked in his ear and then questioned him. He responded that I knew of the cotton, so she repeated the test again showing the same results as the day before, a slight sensorineural hearing loss. The patient left the audiologist with his chart and results right after the test, but somehow never made it back to my office.

The staff and I felt good that we had picked up this malingerer. We all laughed as we thought of him being too embarrassed to come back. Wouldn't you know it, Mr. Blake returned later that afternoon. He raced into the office and threw the chart on the receptionist's desk and ran out again. He must have been scared about stealing a medical chart, even though he was fine with ripping off his company. Anyway, the chart was complete except for one missing item – the audiogram.

Oh what a tangled web we weave when first we practice to deceive! ✚

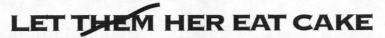

LET ~~THEM~~ HER EAT CAKE

This morning's consult, admitted for nausea and vomiting (*resolved on admission*), was now having severe headaches and low back pain. She weighs at least 400 pounds and brought her own quilt with her. There had a subclavian line inserted for IV access (*hats off to whoever did that*). At lunch time, I walked in and she was lying flat on her back with a plate of cake on her chest, shoveling it over her chin.
A Kodak moment.

It was her quote that made me truly ponder what we do:

"I had to go to eight different ERs before someone would admit me."

✚

As a family practitioner, I see infants as well as adults. Occasionally a mother of one of our kids will deposit a stinky diaper in the trash can in the exam room. You know it as soon as you walk in the room and just deal with it like it's nothing new.

One day I grabbed the chart from the door and entered the room of a new patient without looking at the reason for his visit. Upon entering, the smell of baby poop was overwhelming and I apologized profusely while rooting around in the garbage can searching for the offensive diaper.

Surprised when I found none, I surmised and explained that the nurse had been in the room and had taken the stinker, but that the smell had lingered. The patient to this point had said nothing.

I finally sat down opened his chart and asked, *"So what brings you here today?"*

"The people at work say my feet smell."

✚

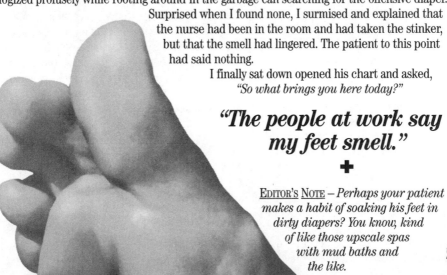

EDITOR'S NOTE – *Perhaps your patient makes a habit of soaking his feet in dirty diapers? You know, kind of like those upscale spas with mud baths and the like.*

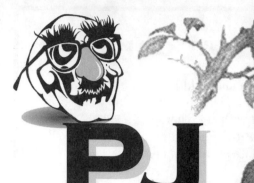

PJ

AND A BARREL OF
MONKEYS

We have all heard about trying to *"get the monkey off your back."* It is an overused cliché in sports. In medicine, we need to investigate this phrase a little more closely. These "monkeys" are actually issues or problems. Patients come into our office with these monkeys all the time. They don't have just one of them either. Many times they have a barrel of monkeys and they want the physician to take them.

I don't know about you, but I am sick of being the zookeeper.

When such patients arrive, they have the monkeys well hidden. Other patients in the waiting room hardly notice. The front staff is usually oblivious to them. Your nurse, however, usually gets a whiff of them. She senses that there are monkeys about. By the time the patient enters the room, their monkeys are all over the place. As soon as you walk in, you realize that the place is a menagerie.

These patients live with these monkeys all the time. They feed them. They take care of them. Now, since you are the doctor, they think they can just hand them over.

It starts with a list.

Complaints of dizziness, fatigue, or headaches are just little monkeys that got the patient to come in. Pretty soon the big monkeys come out. You may know them as depression, situational anxiety, or polysubstance abuse.

There are a lot more monkeys I could name but does it really make a difference. You get the point.

For some reason, these patients think that you deserve their monkeys. They don't want to take care of them anymore. They are tired of them. Their monkeys weigh them down and since they don't want to deal with the issues themselves, they are kind enough to let you do it.

I want to be the first to say, *"I don't want your damn monkeys!"* I've got enough monkeys of my own. It took me a while in private practice to realize that each time I left a patient's room, I had one, two, or three monkeys on my back. The patient would say things like, *"I want you to get me to quit smoking"* or *"I have no energy and I want you to address that."* Other bombshells of relationship problems, run-ins with the law, or problems with money got laid on my back. These monkeys were all over me by the end of the day. I was becoming the **Quasimodo of Medicine**. Sure, the patient felt better, but I was getting burned out feeding all the monkeys they'd left with me.

My answer to this quandary is to turn the tables on the patients.

You must make them take responsibility for their own monkeys. They have to kill the damn things before they make a mess everywhere. Give them assignments to fulfill. Make them jump productive hurdles that will get them to the right place and without a monkey in sight. They need to show some accountability to you because the next time they come in, you will ask them if they followed through. When they say no, you can end the visit and walk out monkey-free.

This is the bottom line –
Either they kill their own monkeys
(or at least show some effort trying to)
or they take their pets somewhere else.

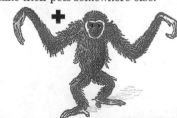

146

BRIGHT IDEA ONE

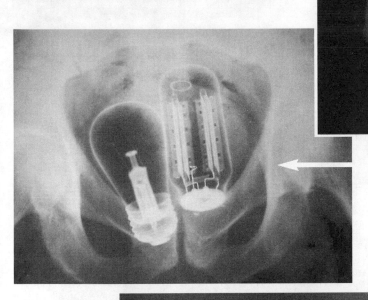

BRIGHT IDEA TWO

QUESTION:
Does it make this idea
twice as bright?

X-Ray Files

NOT SO BRIGHT

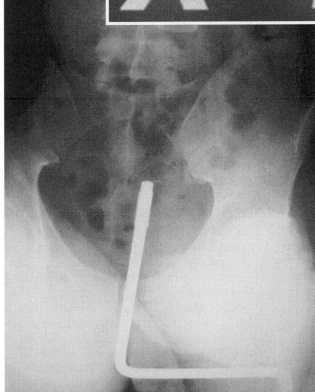

The story is that the man
was painting and "fell" off
the ladder he was using,
landing onto the paintbrush
roller. However, the plot
thickens... he must have
been painting in the nude
because there were no
undergarments between the
paintbrush roller and his
rectal orifice.

*Could he possibly have
made the whole story up?
Inquiring minds want
to know.*

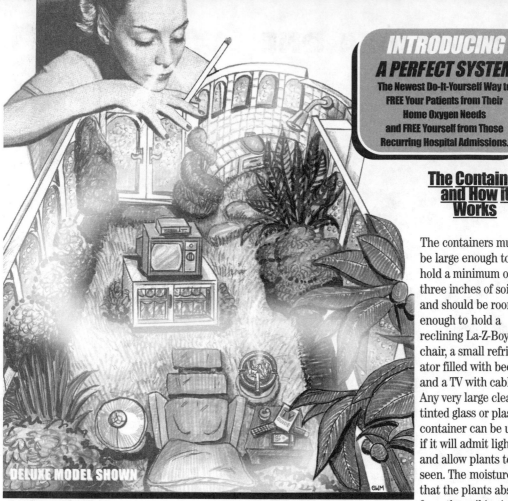

INTRODUCING
A PERFECT SYSTEM
The Newest Do-It-Yourself Way to
FREE Your Patients from Their
Home Oxygen Needs
and FREE Yourself from Those
Recurring Hospital Admissions.

DELUXE MODEL SHOWN

GWM

The Container and How it Works

The containers must be large enough to hold a minimum of three inches of soil and should be roomy enough to hold a reclining La-Z-Boy chair, a small refrigerator filled with beer, and a TV with cable. Any very large clear or tinted glass or plastic container can be used if it will admit light and allow plants to be seen. The moisture that the plants absorb from the soil is given off through the leaves by the process of transpiration. This condenses on the container walls and runs down to moisten the soil again. The atmosphere also remains balanced through the combined plant processes of photosynthesis and respiration. A well-constructed terrarium requires only light and warmth to flourish.

Choice of Plants

The arrangement of the plants within the **COPD Terrarium** should be determined before putting your patient inside. The physician should trace the shape of the container onto a piece of paper and arrange the potted plants to test possible arrangements for optimal CO_2 and O_2 transfer. A regular ceiling fan can be used for air circulation. Most plants recommended for terrariums are moisture-loving types which never become large. Because most houseplants are of tropical or subtropical origin, they thrive in the **COPD Terrarium** environment. Correct selection of the plants to be

A **COPD Terrarium** is a collection of both plants and *Lungers* living in a single container, one that is completely enclosed. These gardens are an excellent place to grow plants, which require a high degree of humidity, and "COPDers" who produce so much extra of that pesky CO_2. Together they will live in complete symbiosis; freeing your patients of their home oxygen needs and you from those recurring hospital admissions.

COPD Terrariums are fun and only require a minimum of care if they are kept sealed. They usually demand little attention and will grow successfully on their own for several months or even years. Regular input of food for the *Lungers*, as well as a TV guide now and then, is all the hassle you will get.

The following is a list of what is required to create your own **COPD Terrarium**:

Constructing & Maintaining Your Own Homemade
COPD Terrarium

incorporated into the garden is vital to its longevity. Since your patients with emphysema have little more than blebs for lungs, small plants of varieties that do not grow quickly are the best choice. Plants of assorted growth habits create a natural landscape, and the garden may be structured from the viewer's point of view. Do not obstruct the TV screen of your patient or they will become irritated if not violent.

Choice of Lungers

We recommend using those patients with a CO^2 greater than 70 mmHg. They seem to blend in well with your new agricultural environment. Be careful to not put more than two *Lungers* in the same **COPD Terrarium**. Many times they will fight which will cause an excessive use of the plant-produced O^2. Since some *Lungers* are also bitter and depressed people, the chance of having two get along are very small. Do not risk the wrong combination!

Planting

You may wish to create a landscape effect by making the plants and soil look like a normal living room. Different types of grass can be used to give a carpet effect.

Avoid clutter as this may confuse your *Lunger*. Often the simpler arrangements, which make use of a few well-placed, attractive plants are much more pleasing to the eye than miniature jungles which appear about to burst through the glass.

Watering

Well-constructed **COPD Terrariums** do not need to be watered because plants recycle the moisture they use. *Lungers* do not recycle their fluids so an emphasis on beer and coffee is needed. A completely enclosed

terrarium requires little or no extra watering. Your *Lunger*, however, may need a shower now and then.

Sunlight and Fertilizer

Do not forget the importance of sunlight for both the plants and the *Lungers*. The former needs it to grow and the latter needs it to stave off Seasonal Affective Disorder.

Fertilizer is also very important but with the new and improved **FECAL-IZER**, your patient's stool can be your plants' best friend.

Cigarettes

This is the beauty of the **COPD Terrarium**. How many times have you seen your patients blow their faces off because they smoke while on home oxygen? There is no chance of combustion in the **COPD Terrarium**. Now your *Lungers* can grow their own tobacco right at home – and smoke it too! *Bad for their health you say?* With such little lung tissue left, does it really matter anymore if they smoke? And that's not all! The **COPD Terrarium** is actually self-regulating. The more the patient smokes the more oxygen they use. Over-users will choke and pass out and the plants will just replenish the oxygen once again until they wake up. No one gets hurt. ✚

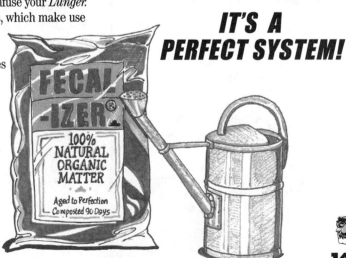

IT'S A PERFECT SYSTEM!

149

LIST OF BAD PROGNOSTIC SIGNS

Medicare patient under 60 who is not in a wheelchair or has a seeing-eye dog

Any adult patient who is accompanied by their mother

Any female patient with migraines who is accompanied by her husband

More than ten drug allergies

Non-anatomic sensory or motor loss (e.g., entire leg)

Pending litigation

Refuses to undergo a test or procedure where the co-pay is more than the cost of a new DVD player because it's too expensive

Work-related injury

ROS (review of systems) more than 50 percent positive

Family members start arguing amongst themselves about patient's illness

Cancels follow-up appointment because doctor would not prescribe pain pills, sleeping medication, or tranquilizers at initial visit. (*Actually, this is a sort of a good sign.*)

Patient is in any position other than sitting or standing when doctor enters the room

Patient has turned off the lights in the exam room or is wearing sunglasses indoors because of photophobia ✚

ANSWERING SERVICE TIPS

BEEP!

My instructions to the answering service for our pain clinic have changed. The first question they were supposed to ask was, *"Is this a medical emergency?"*

It was a trick question. If the answer was yes, then they were told to go to the emergency room. If no, then they were told to call back in the morning. You see, either way, I was not involved.

BEEP!

Here is the problem. The answering service people find this too complicated and subsequently let calls go through. An example would be 1 a.m. last night when a guy called because his intrathecal pump was beeping. (*"Oh I'm so glad you called! They start beeping right before they explode. It has nothing to do with the fact the low reservoir alarm is due to go off today, and you have an appointment in 11 hours to have a pump refill!"*)

BEEP!

BEEP!

Anyway, we changed our system. The new "first question" for the answering service is, *"Do you have any f#cking idea what time it is?"*

I can't believe it took me 23 years to figure that out. ✚

EDITOR'S NOTE - *This may work so well that it could spread like wildfire or they will take away your license. Either way, good luck!*

BEEP!

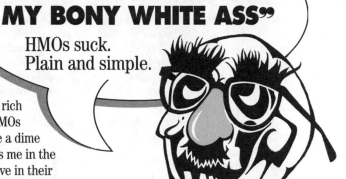

PJ EXPLAINS
"WHY HMOs CAN KISS MY BONY WHITE ASS"

HMOs suck.
Plain and simple.

They do very little for anyone but their stockholders. If I was smart enough and had had the money to invest in them fifteen years ago, I would be rich and I wouldn't be writing about HMOs today. Unfortunately, I didn't make a dime by buying their stock and that puts me in the precarious situation of having to live in their world. I am also bitter about the missed opportunity.

HMOs do not help me.

Let's do a little math problem. Pretend you are taking the SATs all over again. Your first problem is as follows:

You are a family doctor who has to take $12 per member per month. If your patients and their employers are paying approximately $1,000 per family member per year and you have 2,000 patients in your panel, you would be making a whole lot of coin if it was all going to you. Check One: You should

- ❏ Enjoy medicine again
- ❏ See fewer patients in a day and spend more time with them.
- ❏ Stop seeing your therapist for burnout
- ❏ See your family again
- ❏ All of the above

By using the calculations above, you gross $144 per patient per year or $288,000. That is before overhead and doesn't include Medicaid or the freebees of self-pay. Is that:

- ❏ Good   ❏ Bad   ❏ Ugly

The HMOs, on the other hand, get $2 million. Take away what they pay you, and they receive more than $1.7 million. Do you think all that goes to:

- ❏ Labs?   ❏ Medicines?
- ❏ Hospitalizations? ❏ Specialists?
- ❏ Procedures?   ❏ Administrative costs?
- ❏ CEO bonuses? ($40 million on average)

Answer key: You get my point.

HMOs do not help me.
HMOs do not help my patients. *Or my patience.*

The way they bank on people not using their product is perverse in a way. It is kind of like a big health club that banks on its members not showing up and eventually quitting. If everybody showed up to the gym, it would be a mother of a sardine can. It's the same way with HMOs. When people do use their product they block as much as they can. The doctors don't want the patients there because they were paid already. The HMOs don't want referrals (and neither do the physicians) because it comes out of their pockets. HMOs also try to block every procedure, test, or medication they can. My patient can't have Celebrex without a pre-authorization and their first born. My patient can't have an MRI unless the tumor truly causes grand mal seizures because petit mal seizures are, after all, pretty subtle. I exaggerate a bit – or do I?

HMOs do not help my patients. Doctors do.
"AND HMOs CA KISS MY BONY WHITE ASS."

BLACK LESIONS

I was the local hospice's medical director, and as such, was responsible for providing comfort care to the terminally ill, often without direct interaction with the patient. Instead, it is often the case that the nursing and psychosocial staff become my only eyes and ears on the case, apart from the referring physician or any family who I may have encountered outside of the home setting. It is neither necessary nor possible to have seen new patients when they are initially presented to the hospice interdisciplinary team at the weekly meeting and intake rounds.

Cathy was an experienced hospice nurse who was presenting a new hospice referral thought to have severe diabetic peripheral ascular insufficiency, especially in a leg that was being called gangrenous for which only amputation was possible, but was being refused by the patient. Such patients would presumably die of septicemia within days to weeks barring surgical intervention, and since surgery had been barred as an alternative, the patient was probably appropriate for hospice care.

Assessing for appropriateness of a candidate or recent admission to hospice can be done vicariously by the medical director in such a case, as long as it is wet (purulent) gangrene and not just digital infarction without bacterial infection, so-called dry gangrene, characterized by distal blackening of the digits in the absence of pus, gas, or odor. Cathy's description of the limb in question had been unclear, and I was uncertain that the patient had either lesion after her jumbled presentation that alluded to dark coloration of the dorsum of the foot.

"Was the area dark or black?" I asked.

"Black," was the reply.

"Is the foot black on the toes, too?" I followed, assuming that ischemic or embolic infarction could not spare the toes and therefore needed to be present to accept the diagnosis of gangrene, wet or dry.

"Yes, the toes, too."

"How far up does the blackness extend? Does it include the heel or ankle as well?" I asked.

"Yes. The whole leg is black. Both legs are completely black except for the soles of the feet," Cathy offered.

Now I was very confused. This didn't sound like gangrene, and if it wasn't, the patient may have had six or more months of natural life remaining, a disqualifying factor in most cases when judging initial hospice admission appropriateness. I was beginning to sense that I was going to have to lay eyes on the "lesion" myself. But what could Cathy be describing?

"I'm stumped," I admitted. *"I don't know what makes both legs black but spares the soles."*

"Her hands are the same," said Cathy. *"The whole body is black. Did I mention that she was African-American?"*

No. Nice presentation, I thought. The patient was discharged. Being black is not a terminal diagnosis, even in Missouri.

BLACK PHLEGM

From there, I made my hospital rounds to see my new internal medicine admissions. One was a gentleman who was admitted with post-traumatic, lower extremity deep vein thrombosis, chest pain, and productive cough. Suspecting pulmonary embolism and perhaps infarction as well, I asked Ron if his mucous contained any blood or red discoloration. *"No, but it's dappled with black flecks,"* he stated.

What now? I thought. Incidentally, Ron was white, so these weren't pieces of himself that he was coughing up. At least, not melanotic pieces. Once bitten, twice shy I thought, still reeling from the bizarre events of hospice rounds earlier in the morning. No coal history. What else gives black color to sputum if not necrotic tissue? Blood is never darker than maroon in phlegm. I was stumped again by a history of atypical black discoloration.

I returned to see this same patient that evening while rounding again, and Ron informed me that he had saved me a specimen of his blackened mucus in a tissue on the bed stand. I unwadded the mess and peered at the contents within. Bright red blood. Garden variety hemoptysis.

"Does this look black to you?" I queried in amazement.

"Yeah, it does, Doc. I'm color blind."

My fault. I forgot to ask this man what his complete chromic visual spectrum was, and I slackened on the physical exam, having omitted the Ishihara color vision test required by Mediocre, er, Medicare, to qualify for the coveted 99223 reward (code for average office visit bill): thorough. *Boy, was I feeling stupid.* Color me red – or, black in the eyes of some. ✚

Sure you have diabetes.
Sure it is going to kill you.
Heck, you have to die from something, don't you?

PJ Pharmaceuticals understands your dilemma.

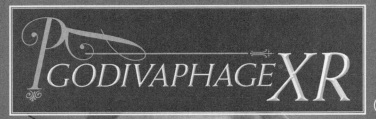

®

With *GODIVAPHAGE XR®* you can have your cake and eat it too. *Literally!* Each ball contains four ounces of the best chocolate this side of Switzerland. Oh yeah, it also has 500 mg of Metformin inside. *Talk about a spoon full of sugar making the medicine go down!* Sit down after a nice meal and enjoy one or two balls of *GODIVAPHAGE XR®* after dinner and get your sugar under pretty good control. *We guarantee you won't forget your medicine now!**

**Taking one too many balls of GODIVAPHAGE XR® may lead to hypoglycemia and death. Keep locked away from children as they are sure to crash and burn with just one of these puppies.*

Those highfalutin doctors talk about dieting. It's not that easy to eat right when you're hungry. Now these physicians in those fancy white jackets tell us that smoking is bad for us! Why don't they make up their minds? We all know that stopping smoking just makes us eat more.

PJ PHARMACEUTICALS
The Realistic Drug Company
©2002 PJP

STAND UP! QUICK!

I fondly recall the time that two other anesthesia attendings and I were walking out to the parking lot along with one of the residents. We saw a guy collapse on the corner and rushed over. We all knelt over him. One of us said, *"I think he isn't breathing."*

At that point, reaching deep down into our collective wisdom and experience as board-certified anesthesiologists (I also have fellowship training in critical care), and with lightning-like reflexes, all three of the attendings, myself included, stood up as fast as we could. This left the resident kneeling on the ground next to the apneic man.

We all stared at him expectantly. **Like a fraternity pledge swallowing a goldfish, he dutifully started mouth-to-mouth on the stricken man, who promptly vomited all over the place.** *We're talking Old Faithful here!* The resident started gagging and retching. Naturally, we stepped in to help by using the man's coat to wipe off the vomit so the resident could continue his life-saving maneuvers.

We got the man over to the ER, where unfortunately he later died. As "Thoughtful Attendings," in gratitude to this heroic resident who performed such a selfless and nauseating act, we remembered to ask the ER staff to send off serology for communicable diseases, which was negative.

You can confirm this independently by contacting a renowned attending at Duke, who was the resident. I'm sure he will enjoy reliving the experience. ✚

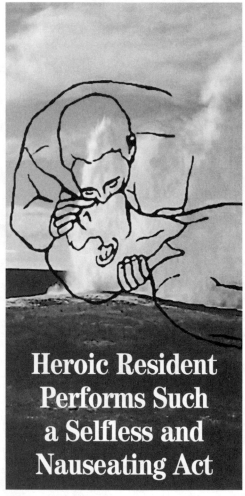

Heroic Resident Performs Such a Selfless and Nauseating Act

Here are some reasons given for requested radiology studies. Sometimes they are the study that was ordered. I will give you our interpretation in parentheses when I think you may need it.

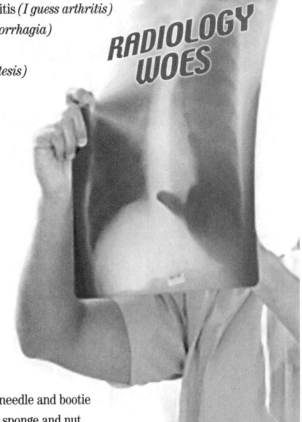

Reason for Study for Chest X-ray: SOB/Resent Cabbage

Reason for Study for Chest X-ray: Failure to Breathe

Reason for Cspine X-ray: R/O Oreochitis *(I guess arthritis)*

Ballistic Metastases Metrogagia *(Menorrhagia)*

We Need It

Post Thorus Synthesis *(post thoracentesis)*

Mummer *(murmur)*

Pre-op RED ALERT

Injured Groins while tightroping

Patient known to you

Tub placement

Assault with high heels

Left total lip replacement

Stag Wound to Chest

R/O Lung Absence

Weightless

Shot with Taser by SWAT team

R/O Phewmonia

Allergic to "red food"

S/P Chest Ache Removal

Shortness of Breast

OR S/P Post liver transplant, missing needle and bootie

OR S/P Post-op nephrectomy, missing sponge and nut

Face Vs. Ground *(I guess the patient lost that battle)*

For L-S spine series: Pt. c/o pain with radiation
    (Time to stop ordering X-rays)

Reason for CT Brain: Mass in chest – to see if it has climbed up
    into the brain

R/O Os Good Shlottess Disease *(and a similar one)* R/O Oscar Shlatters

Lumbar spine with erect penis *(Lumbar spine with erect pelvis)*

Reason for Cerebral Angiogram: R/O Subarachnoid Hemorrhoids

Reason for Pregnancy Ultrasound: Spootin *(Can't even guess on this one)*

Anal X-ray *(Annual X-ray)*

Reproductive chest pain *(Bummer!)*

"End of Life" Mode ✚

Learn to Talk
ADMINISTRALIAN
The Complete Interactive Learning Solution

#1 ADMINISTRALIAN SOFTWARE PROGRAM
Personalized Learning System: Version 3.0
• 4 CD Set • Adjustable Study Plan

Learn to Talk ADMINISTRALIAN offers a complete, in-depth learning system to achieve all around fluency on how to blow smoke up people's asses.
Unique real-world conversation simulations and speech recognition enhance your learning experience as you are able to converse and compare your pronunciation to native speakers and bullshit artists.

Pre-Assessment Test
Subject Specific Study Topics

A dynamic technology that you customize to your study needs, skill level and time constraints.

Download to your PDA and be able to interpret all the garbage others are throwing around the conference room.

DEVELOP COMPREHENSION, READING, AND WRITING SKILLS

ACHIEVE FLUENCY

The best way to learn Administralian is to practice. Try it with your kids. Try it with your staff. You will not believe how much you can fool them. Remember that wise saying, "If you can't fool them with science, then dazzle them with bullshit."
Interactive conversations with administrators and CEOs will enable you to learn from the best. See meaningless hand gestures and fake empathetic facial expressions. Master the art of filibustering. Learn how to promise the world in order to give physicians hope and get them out of your hair.

MASTER WORDS AND PHRASES

OVER 100 LESSONS
including
Vocabulary

Pronunciation

Filibustering

E-mail wizardry to pretend you are still at work

Tall tales for large groups

Writing long-winded and worthless memos

Hiding from doctors

Forming useless committees

Examples of Cultural Nuances

1. Always say the person's name; *("Well, Jim, I believe . . .")* as it makes them feel important.
2. Remember to stroke the physicians frequently and vigorously. They have low self-esteem and are easily flattered.
3. Create the illusion that the problem is always on the front burner *(when you forgot what the problem really was).*
4. Take fake notes when they offer complaints and criticisms *(never tilt the pad down in case they are looking).*
5. Talk incessantly as doctors have a very short attention span and after awhile you will drive them crazy enough to agree to anything.
6. Claim ignorance on a particular topic or situation but say you will get right on top of it.
7. When you find that you are getting in too deep on some topic, use diversionary topics in order to confuse the overwhelmed physician.
8. Use examples of other organizations in order to bore your listeners to tears.
9. Make up data to support your point knowing that no one will ever challenge it.
10. Pledge to create a committee or action group or task force and then find reasons why it never meets.

EXAMPLES OF SOME EASY TRANSLATIONS

ADMINISTRALIAN	PHYSICIAN TRANSLATION
I hear you.	How do I get the hell out of here?
I want to bring this to the larger group (or smaller group.)	I will have forgotten what you told me the minute I leave this room.
I consider you a friend and valued advisor.	I would have fired your lazy ass years ago if I could have found a way to pull it off.
I want to thank you for your honesty.	You sniveling and ungrateful bastard!
I will definitely get back to you on this important topic.	I will bury this crap so far in a pile on my desk that it would take a sniffing dog to find it.
I understand what you are going through.	Now leave me the hell alone!
Your value to this company cannot be underestimated.	Feel better now? Good. Shut-up and sit your ass down.
Your input is extremely important.	You are a moron. Go treat patients and let the real professionals do their job.
You are a leader and innovator for this organization.	You are a royal pain in the ass and everyone in administration hates you.
So correct me if I am wrong but what I hear you saying is . . .	I am saying these empty words in order to fool you into believing that I am listening. I'm not.
Your contributions to the organization are greatly appreciated.	If you died now we would forget you in a minute (who are you again?).
He has moved on to a practice of a better fit.	We got his ass out of here as soon as we discovered his website doing digital rectal exams on himself.
Though his personality may be a little high-strung, his surgical ability is greatly valued.	This guy could be serial killer, for as much as we care, as long as he keeps generating all that fu*king cash!
This new computer system will approve patient care, quality assurance, meet HIPPA guidelines, and help communication in the office while reducing medical errors.	We will fire three of your office help and shift that work to the physician with an extra two hours of computer work a day thereby saving us lots of money and giving it to the CEO.
The benefit of your electronic medical record is easy patient record access at home and on-call.	We just want you to do more work.

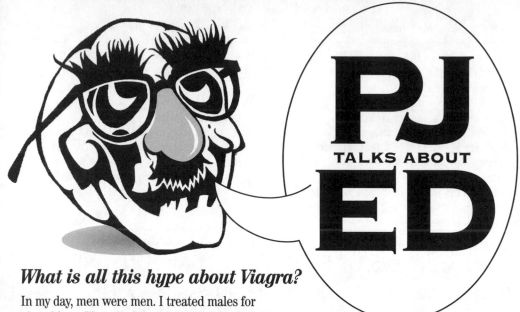

PJ

TALKS ABOUT

ED

What is all this hype about Viagra?

In my day, men were men. I treated males for real problems like a limb hanging off or neuritis. We didn't have all these problems you have now. Now you have male athletes promoting this stuff. *Athletes?!* In my time, the football players didn't even have face masks much less athletic supporters or cups. If they were kicked or bitten on the testicles they would just kick or bite their opponents back.

Now male patients need coddling. They come in for erectile dysfunction. *They don't even call it impotence anymore!* Most of these men already have had kids so I can't figure out what the problem is. These new-fangled questionnaires talk about maintaining erections, stiffness, and arousal ability. *Excuse me?* We didn't care about that back yonder. I had better things to do as a physician than to talk to a patient about the stiffness quality of his Johnson.

I would tell him to get a Popsicle stick and some duct tape and get the hell out of my office.

Now they want endurance for their erections. *Endurance!* What do they care about endurance? Just get in and get out. These youngsters should care less about quality and more about getting finished.

The point is that men these days are thinking more about their penis than ever before. Instead of letting it whither on the vine, patients want their maleness to stand at attention at a moment's notice.

Even worse, they want their doctors to be the accomplices to this unnatural ritual.

I say no! Let your men suffer like we did. Let them sit in their rocking chairs and whittle their sticks (*no pun intended*) reminiscing about the days when their penises actually worked. When Grandpa maintains the ability to have an erection like a 20-year-old, he is not only a danger to himself but Grandma as well. And trust me, you would much rather deal with him than her. ✚

158

Case Records of the Placebo General Hospital

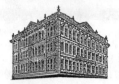

*Primary Care Monthly Pathoclinicosocial
Mental Mastubatory Exercises*

BILL LEFRANCE, M.D.
Internship-trained General Practitioner
CORNELIUS PARODY, M.D.
*Clinical Professor, Placebo University,
Researcher Extraordinaire, and
self-described smart guy*
DR. W. SCOTT WINNIPER, M.D.
*General Adult Psychiatry, subspecializes
in familial MOCUS*
DR. ANNIE SCHMECKL, M.D.
Family Practitioner for over 40 years

Case 11-2002

PRESENTATION OF CASE

A 51-year-old man was seen in the office for recurrent fatigue. The patient had been well up until age 12. He has had progressive feelings of "just not doing well" to the point where he now demands "something be done." Symptoms includes dyspnea which are significant enough that it has made it very hard for him to smoke three packs of cigarettes a day. His dietary habits have changed in that he no longer can eat a full pizza due to early satiety. He now only eats around seven slices. No weight loss has been found. In fact, he has gone up an average of three pants sizes per year since college.

The patient has a constellation of symptoms which include testicular tenderness, a rash under his pannus (folds of abdominal fat), and debilitating backaches (which prevent gainful employment). He also describes abdominal pain which occurs once every four months, lasts up to two full seconds, and makes him feel "funny afterwards." This is usually alleviated with foul-smelling flatulence.

Our patient is a father of seven and divorced thrice. Most of his medical work-up has occurred while in prison and included all procedures that end in –oscopy (cystocopy, endoscopy, colonoscopy, bronchoscopy, arthroscopy). All the patient's labs, except those things that we have no idea what they are, were normal. All review of systems was positive.

On physical exam, the patient appeared well. No abnormalities, as hard as we looked, were found.

DIAGNOSIS DISCUSSION

DR. BILL LEFRANCE – *May we review the studies or procedures?*

DR. CORNELIUS PARODY – *No.*

DR. LEFRANCE – *Why not?*

DR. PARODY – *Because we don't have them. They are still at the prison.*

DR. LEFRANCE– *Well that's a bunch of sh#t!*

DR. PARODY – *Hey, if you don't like it, you can go . . .*

DR. ANNIE SCHMECKL – *Dr. Parody!*

DR. PARODY – *Sorry. Anyone else with some thoughts?*

DR. W. SCOTT WINNIPER – *Obviously, there is a lot less here than meets the eye. I think this is an obvious case of SLS (Shitty Life Syndrome). No treatment is possible.*

DR. SCMECKL – *I agree.*

DR. LEFRANCE – *Well that's good enough for me. Anyone up for lunch then? There are some bagels here.*

DR. WINNIPER – *These bagels suck. They are also stale. How about some Thai food? There's a restaurant around the corner.*

DR. SCHMECKL – *I'm in.*

DR. PARODY – *Me too. Let's make Lefrance pay. That cheap bastard never reaches into his wallet.*

DR. LEFRANCE – *One more word out of you Parody and I am seriously going to kick your ass.*

DR. ANGUS BLACK (suddenly awakens ten minutes later) – *Hey, where did everyone go?* ✚

PRACTICE MANAGEMENT CORNER

Written by Al Truistic B.S.

Hi everyone. I'm Al Truistic B.S. and I am here with some **TIPS ON HOW TO MAKE YOUR PRACTICE HUM.** Sure, I have little experience. Sure, my ideas are "pie in the sky" and make little sense. *Does that really matter?* It doesn't seem to stop other practice management experts from giving their recommendations. **I RECOMMEND YOU START USING HAND SIGNALS TO COMMUNICATE WITH YOUR STAFF. WITH PRACTICE, YOU WILL SAVE PRECIOUS TIME IN THE OFFICE!** Just like a coach using a hand signal to tell the quarterback what play to call, you can use

OFFICIAL PHYSICIAN

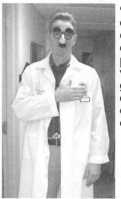
"I need an EKG done on this patient while I go get a cup of coffee."

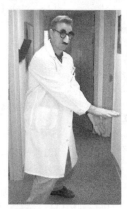
"We need to set up for a Pap smear."

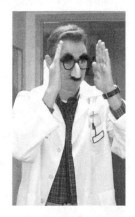

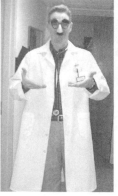
"I will need a chaperone to do a breast exam on this patient."

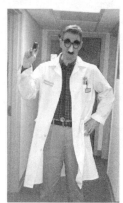
"This patient can talk forever. Wait about 3 minutes and then beep me out with a fake page."

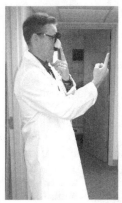

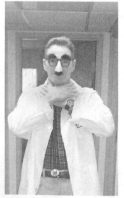
"Tell the drug rep to leave the office now or I will be forced to choke the sh#t out of him."

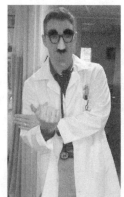
"Do me a favor and grab some Viagra samples for this patient?"

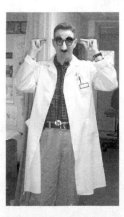

hand signals to tell your nurse or secretary what they need to do.

Sounds stupid? Maybe, but you will thank me when you have an **EXTRA SIX MINUTES OF FREE TIME AT THE END OF THE DAY.** Our model physician shown below is demonstrating some examples that may work for you. You may want to add some new ones.

If you have some signals that you want to donate, just e-mail me at PJ@placebojournal.com

Good luck and win one for the dipper.

HAND SIGNALS

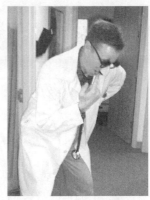

"Do not order me the chicken salad again. It made me want to vomit!"

"Get me the extra large speculum. With the hydraulic jack."

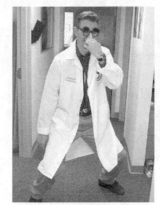

"Dear God, there is a Code Brown in this exam room. Someone get the disinfectant spray."

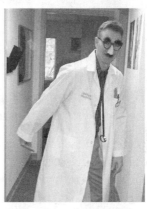

"Have that insurance rep on the phone kiss my fat ass."

"Be careful, this patient is a lawyer. His nose grows every time he speaks."

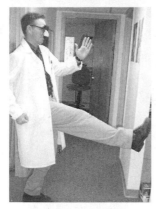

"Tell the patient whatever you want but I am outta here."

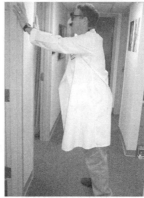

"Nurse, we are out of Vaseline in here."

"I need to get this patient's ears cleaned in here."

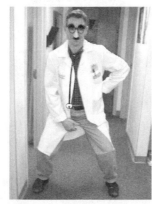

"Do something to help me because this patient is driving me *NUTS!*"

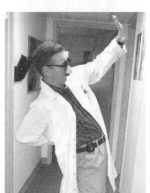

"Stop everything! I really need to move my bowels! *I mean now!*"

From coast to coast, thousands of hopefuls are gathering to get the chance to compete for the crown of the sickest man or woman in America.

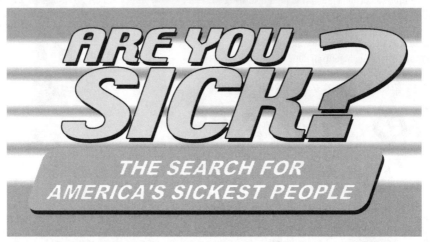

ARE YOU SICK?

THE SEARCH FOR AMERICA'S SICKEST PEOPLE

Finally, they can prove how ill they are and now, on live TV, someone may believe them.

Talent, real disease, and strategy are not allowed; just a deep personal belief that you really feel like sh*t. Now TV viewers get their chance to vote on the Sick Zone. Watch participants from each region sweat, faint, or cry as they face a celebrity panel of experts.

Crisscrossing America for casting calls in many cities and pouring over medical records, the producers divided the country into "Sick Zones" that included every state. Watch this summer as we'll learn who America chooses as really being sick. The process of elimination will continue each week until one breathless man and one aching woman are crowned as . . .

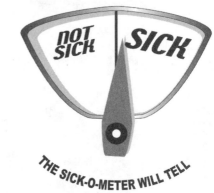

THE SICK-O-METER WILL TELL

AMERICA'S SICKEST PEOPLE

No real diseases are allowed. Only those people who believe they are sick but without a true diagnosis are included. Designer diseases such as irritable bowel syndrome, chronic fatigue syndrome, multiple chemical sensitivity syndrome, adult attention deficit disorder, and fibromyalgia are not only acceptable but encouraged!

Only on

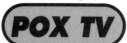

POX TV

The only station that would sell its kidney for better ratings.

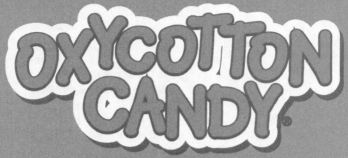
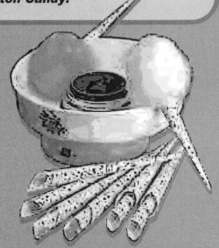
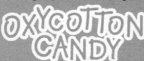

1 Don't try a new drug on a patient until it has been on the market for one year. For your family, wait five years.

2 A test was unnecessary if it turns out normal. But are you going to complain?

3 Some people have a condition called "your number is up."

4 A therapeutic test means that if the treatment works, then maybe you had the right diagnosis, unless, of course, it was some other diagnosis.

5 If the placebo works almost as well as the therapy, then the therapy is not better than the placebo no matter what any statistician says.

6 I challenge anyone to tell when a sore throat is caused by a virus and not a bacterial colony without doing 14 days of tests at the Centers for Disease Control. That's why we older docs give antibiotics. That's also why we don't see cases of acute rheumatic fever anymore.

7 The *Physicians Desk Reference* now has 3,500 pages of 8-point type. I know all the drugs in there in minutest detail except for the one you just asked about.

8 We were taught in medical school to learn only about 20 drugs, but learn them well. Now the doctor should know 500 but he might barely know the names of most of them. Don't tell anybody I said that.

9 I liked better what they said in 1890 when my great grandmother died in childbirth at home. It was God's will. Better than it's the doctor's fault and let's sue.

10 Want to know what to do for grief or depression? Get up every morning, say a blessing that you are still breathing, and go to work.

11 I am just as perplexed about the here-before as I am about the here-after.

12 Socrates had a theory that the soul knew everything before it was born, then forgot; his job was to ask questions of people till they remembered what they had always known.

13 I'm trying to learn everything there is to know and I am almost finished.

14 Osler, the great physician, was not incensed when someone failed to follow his instructions. He said, now we will find out which one of us is wrong.

15 Fifty years ago we dispensed a lot of placebos. There were green and pink pills, pink and chocolate aspirins, and Caripeptic liquid which smelled and looked like tar. Now I don't know any doctor who dispenses or uses placebos. Now you can get all the quack medicines you want at the health food store.

16 There were and are pure placebos and impure placebos. Sugar is a pure placebo. Aspirin is an impure placebo because it actually does something.

17 I once asked a health food store owner if the whole bran she was selling was pasteurized and if she knew how many rat droppings or mouse hairs the FDA allowed in that product. She thought a minute, then proudly replied that any rat or mouse that was eating that stuff was therefore healthy and not to worry.

18 I don't know if you know this, but doctors joke around a lot while they are operating on you. We once had an anesthesiologist who used to say "this patient is ruined; get me a new one." People like their doctors to have a sense of humor.

19 Or how about this: what should the doctor do if the patient walks out of the office and drops dead in the hallway? Call 911? No. First he should turn the patient around so it looks as if he had been coming in. Sorry; I can't resist sick jokes.

20 Are you sure you want a complete checkup? In the old days, a complete physical examination included an exploratory abdominal operation, burring holes in your head, a spinal tap, bronchoscopy, sigmoidoscopy, and gastroscopy. A complete exam was fatal. ✚

X-Ray Files

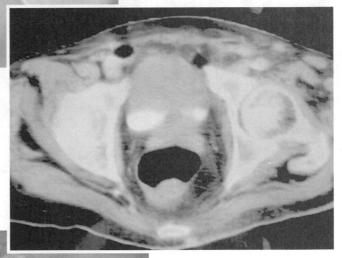

" *I'm allergic to NUTS, but I will take a BOLT.* **"**

" DOH!"

Homer Simpson shows up in a pelvic CT

" Look! Up in the sky! It's a bird, It's a plane... **"**

Nope, it's a bird, as seen in a duodenum UGI

165

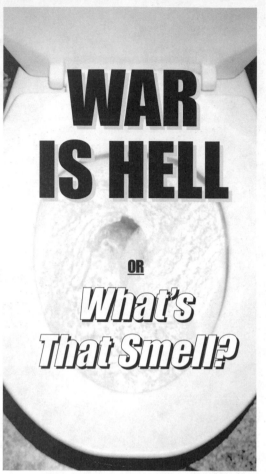

WAR IS HELL

OR

What's That Smell?

She was pure as snow. As she entered the exam room, it was if she was floating on air. My angelic 80-year-old patient was one of my all-time favorite customers. She was sweet and kind. She reminded me of the sweet little old lady in the Sylvester and Tweety bird cartoons. Little did I know the evil that lurked inside.

The exam went smooth as silk. I dealt with her issues professionally and expeditiously. She was alert and enjoyable to talk to. Her mind was sharp as a tack. As she left, I thought to myself, *"I wish I had more patients like Meg."*

That is when all hell broke loose.

Meg decided to turn left into the bathroom near my exit sign. No one knew she was in there. We did know, however, when she left. The rest of the story can only be explained in military terms.

It was as if a weapon of mass destruction had been unleashed. By the time we all noticed, Meg was long gone. I ran out of my office and began questioning my people. Assessment of damage is always the first protocol. *"Lisa, what the hell is that smell!!!"*

Even with our brains a little foggy, we figured it out quite quickly. Ground Zero was my bathroom. Immediately, I shouted out orders to my troops (just like in real battles, the generals never go near the front).

Coincidentally, I just finished watching my favorite war series of all time, *Band of Brothers*, for the second time. Subsequently, my orders were eerily similar to those of Captain Winters. I would say things like, *"Get in there!!"* or *"Go, go, go"* or *"Hang tough"* or *"Keep shooting* (the disinfectant spray)! *Don't let up!"*

When I felt the enemy was neutralized, I walked into the bathroom to inspect the results. Just like the general who walks onto the battlefield after the battle is over, I looked things over as my staff beamed with pride.

That is when I saw it.
On the floor was a brown streak.
Dear God, we had a contamination breach!! I looked at Lisa with horror as I scrambled to save myself (leaving everyone else behind). My staff could hear me bark orders as I ran away (again just like a real general would).

Luckily, Lisa came into my office and informed me that is was just remnants of dirt from Meg's shoe. The war was over. We could finally rest. Meg is home now and probably laughing to herself about her misgivings. For us, we will live on. We will go on knowing that some battles will always be fought because there never will be a winner. We are fighting ourselves and that struggle is a microcosm of… Sorry, it got away from me. Battle fatigue, you know.

Let me sum this up by saying,

WAR IS HELL. +

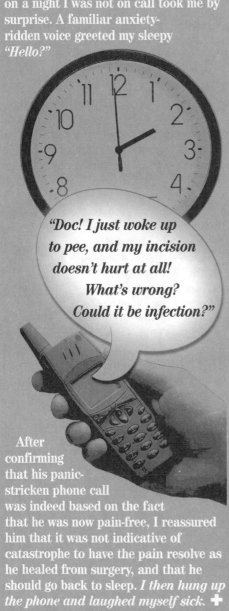

Hernia repair patients tend to be anxious in the first week or two following surgery (something about that phrase "testicular loss" that one mentions during the informed consent, perhaps).

One particularly nervous gentleman called me almost daily for concerns ranging from a "fever" of 98.9 to the small amount of swelling associated with the body's reaction to the Dexon skin closure. Still, the 2 a.m. phone call at home on a night I was not on call took me by surprise. A familiar anxiety-ridden voice greeted my sleepy *"Hello?"*

"Doc! I just woke up to pee, and my incision doesn't hurt at all! What's wrong? Could it be infection?"

After confirming that his panic-stricken phone call was indeed based on the fact that he was now pain-free, I reassured him that it was not indicative of catastrophe to have the pain resolve as he healed from surgery, and that he should go back to sleep. *I then hung up the phone and laughed myself sick.* ✚

DUCT TAPE

While providing care in the Family Practice Clinic at a North Carolina Marine Corps Base Naval Hospital, Mrs. LeJeune Grunt, a female in her late 50s, presented with complaints of nocturnal pruritis ani (rectal itching) for several weeks. She lived in a somewhat rural area with her husband and various other animals and I surmised that she probably had enterobius (parasitic) infestation. However, not seeing any midday laggers in the anal verge or in the crypts, I was curious as to what might be found on a "Scotch tape" prep. I gave her a paper bag containing three of four glass slides and advised her about using cellophane tape at the time of the actual "itching" and returning at least two "good slide specimens" to me on a walk-in basis.

Two days later, the clinic nurse notified me that there was a "lady with a paper bag for me to check." I replied that I knew who it was and that she should give me the bag and let the patient have a seat. I took the bag into our procedure room to view the slides under a microscope. It was difficult to stifle a loud guffaw (*I was unsuccessful*). You see, inside the bag, were two slides covered with silver duct tape, several pubic hairs protruding and a note which read, *"My husband couldn't find any Scotch tape last night, so he used this. I hope it will be okay."* I debated as to whether or not to ask her to redo this procedure, but then thought, if her itching was so intense she could endure this "take home lab test" then she must have pinworms and had earned her treatment. After 100 mg of mebendazole and a follow up one week later, she was symptom free. I am not sure if it was the antihelminthic or the duct tape treatment which effected the cure, but I will keep the duct tape in mind if antihelminthics do not prove successful. ✚

Diary of a New Pharmaceutical

WEEK ONE I can't believe that right out of college, a Fortune 500 company has hired me! My major in Biology and minor in Elizabethan Poetry sure must have helped. I think the fact that I was the head cheerleader in college proved my abundance of team spirit. To be making $50,000 a year at age 23 isn't too shabby. And I get a new car, too!

WEEK TWO My bosses seem really nice. I haven't met anyone else out in the field yet. Got a lot of information to study before training starts. There is a lot to know about hypertension, I'll tell you that. It is so interesting to learn how each mechanism of how our drug works. I wonder why they even need sales reps when it is obvious that our ACE inhibitor is the best. The information they have given me to look at shows how it so superior to the competitors. This job is going to be a piece of cake! I bet the doctors are going to love seeing me come their way.

WEEK FOUR Boy, those tests were hard, but I passed all of them. Going to Florida for a big company meeting. This is awesome. A free trip to Orlando. Theme parks. Meeting other reps from around the country. There are a lot of other pharmaceutical reps that were cheerleaders. That's weird.

WEEK FIVE The meetings were inspiring! There were thousands of us chanting our company name! The lectures on our products just proved I picked the best team to join. There is no question we possess the most effective and unique products available. I can see myself working for this company forever. Nothing is going to stop me from climbing their ladder to a higher administrative level.

WEEK SEVEN Another field rep had me shadow him for a day. He seemed a little down when I met him; however, he seemed to perk up once he saw me. I am sure it is a pick-me-up for him to mentor someone new. He kept asking me

168

why I would pick this job. Then he asked if I can handle personal rejection. Of course I can handle rejection. I remember when I didn't get picked for junior prom queen. I cried for weeks but I eventually got over it and became stronger in the long run. Most of our day was spent on the road talking or trying to get into different medical offices. We only got to meet two doctors. *Boy, were they in a rush!* I don't think the field rep did such a great job. Our product is so good, he needs to get right in those doctors' faces! I can't wait until it is my turn.

WEEK EIGHT First day by myself. Met Dr. Smith. He must be stressed because he cut me off in the middle of my sentence and walked away. He must have forgotten I was there because he never came back. Dr. Johnson was just the opposite. It was great. It seemed he wouldn't stop talking to me. In fact, he wanted to meet me for dinner to just talk about my drug. What was really funny is that he forgot what drug I even had but promised he would use it no matter what is is. I am one hell of a salesperson!

MONTH THREE I am not sure why some doctors won't even meet with me. They want some samples but that is all. Had a lunch with a group of internists. They didn't even show up and I spent $200 on lunch for their staff. They weren't even that thankful either. That was kind of rude.

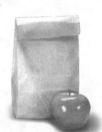

MONTH FOUR Still having trouble getting in to see some doctors. Dr. Ryan told me off and was extremely irritable. He said I was too forceful. I sat in my car and cried for a half-hour. I know I can do better at this. I think our drug is pretty good. I just need to be more assertive.

MONTH FIVE Rode with my boss, who watched my every move. I was really nervous. Still couldn't get in to some offices. What was worse was that my boss kept interrupting me like he was making the sale himself. *Listen, buddy, if you want my job you can have it.* When he left I cried in my car for 15 minutes.

MONTH SIX Had another dinner program for doctors. Only a few showed. The speaker wanted his

Representative (aka Drug Rep)

money right then and there like I was the one who was paying him out of my own account. Then the mother f$%&^r starting talking positively about our competitors! *Whore.*

MONTH SEVEN The marketing people wanted us to have a "birthday party" for our ACE inhibitor. It has been on the market for three years now and they recommend we use the birthday hats and napkins that they gave us. It has our logo and drug name on it. They said the doctors would love it. *Who the f%&^ are they kidding?* As if I am going to get the few doctors that even give me the time of day to light candles and wear hats because our lousy "me too" drug is three years old and selling like sh&*? *Do these marketing people even know what's going on out in the real world?*

MONTH EIGHT Dr. Smith, who was so rude to me, wants to know if I have any baseball tickets for the upcoming series. *I wonder if the phrase "kiss my ass" means anything to him.* Saw Dr. Johnson recently. After the "episode" which occurred at our last dinner, I have purposely stayed away from him. The restraining order still remains. He needs to get a life.

MONTH NINE Went back to our bullsh&% meeting in Florida again. Who are they fooling with this AMWAY crap? This is all cult worship anyway. *In fact, I'd rather drink Kool-Aid laced with cyanide than sell this piece of sh$& drug.* We met in small groups and they tried to teach us new points that would convince any doctor to use our drug. Talk about a circle jerk. Got drunk most nights I was down there.

MONTH TEN The company is getting on my case more and more. They want to know what I am doing every minute of every day. They want signatures. They want programs. They want my first-born. My boss is a prick and if he interrupts me one more time I am going to kick him in his balls.

MONTH ELEVEN Slept with Dr. Johnson. Fu$# it, I needed the numbers. I am also giving away stocking stuffers of goodies to any doctor that will write my loser medication. Whatever it takes to make

bonus. Dr. Flock again tells me he is writing our drug. *What a fu*^%g liar.* We buy the prescription numbers right from the pharmacy so I know what his numbers actually are and this guy bullsh%ts me right to my face. I think he wants to sleep with me.

MONTH TWELVE Slept with my boss. I needed to keep him off my case. One more dinner program and I will put the cyanide in the doctors' drinks myself. Every time I get new marketing material, I throw it right in the trash. *Our company sucks.* I know I hit all numbers but they changed the threshold at the last minute and screwed me out of my bonus.

MONTH THIRTEEN *This job sucks.* If I see another pompous physician I will kick him right in the balls like I did my boss. I will die before I ever feed a bunch of overweight and ungrateful staff workers again. Told my boss to go screw himself or screw Dr. Johnson and leave me the f&^k alone. Threw my keys to the generic minivan at him and walked away with my pride. Never again will I work for a pharmaceutical company.

MONTH FIFTEEN Took a job at our rival. They got some new stuff in the pipeline. The money is even better than my old company. Called Dr. Johnson, meeting him Tuesday night. ✚

What is so wrong about cigarettes anyway?

Our good friends at the tobacco companies care about their customers. Why would they want to hurt them?

SMOKE 'EM IF YOU GOT 'EM

Sure their product eventually kills them, but is that so wrong?

One would think that making a product that shortens the life span of their customers would be a poor strategy. Not true. Let's give these companies their due. They came up with a brilliant business plan that others thought would fail. Well, it didn't and now others follow in their path. Some pharmaceutical companies and automotive companies have shown that even though they may be peddling a faulty product which kills their customer as well, it doesn't matter that much as long as the profits make up for it. Isn't it the American way – sacrifice a few to gain so much?

I am not here to bash these high profile companies. That is way too easy. Some would say too risky, as I don't want to get my ass sued. Instead, let's focus a little on the smokers of the world. They don't have the fancy lawyers to defend them.

Don't let smokers scare you. Sure, they talk a big a game, but deep inside they are just marshmallows (*shriveled up from all the smoking*). There is nothing better to hear a smoker talk about than being free to do what he or she wants to do.

"I don't want to change my ways."

170

"Let me live doing what I want to do. At least I'll die happy."

"Stop telling me to quit smoking, and fix my cough."

"My uncle lived until 103 years and smoked 13 packs of unfiltered cigarettes a day. What do your medical books say about that?"

These are proud people and are accountable for their own actions.
Who are we kidding?

They are the biggest whiners and wimps that have been put on this great planet. As soon as they are a little sick, they are in your face wanting help. Mention quitting and they are offended and mad at you. Their cigarettes are never the cause for anything, except to the physician. And they are sick of us telling them about it. God forbid they get cancer and everything changes. Then the cigarettes are surely to blame and not them.

Breast cancer patients somehow (and wrongfully) blame themselves for their illness. They question if they should have eaten better or exercised more. *Not smokers.*

No, they are the first ones to say that those damn tobacco companies made them do it. Those evil empires hooked them and they therefore couldn't quit. These same patients have forgotten all the warnings both on the packages as well as the repeated ones given by their doctors. They were innocent and not accountable for this disease, and now there are only two things to do – *sue and keep on smoking.*

I, for one, say leave our friends at the tobacco companies alone. If smokers want help (*they never do*), they will come in for a patch or pill. Then they will fail and start smoking again.

The problem is that without being truly committed (*they never are*), these patients are doomed to failure. Very rarely do we see a smoker really get so motivated that he or she will do what it takes to quit. The rest are still out there blaming those non-smokers for making them go outside in the cold and do their nasty deed. Or they are driving to their lawyer's office, blowing the smoke in their children's faces along the way. To those people, we ask you to give our tobacco comrades some peace so they can do what they do best –

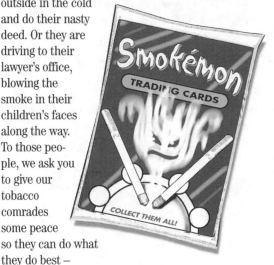

creating better methods to get us addicted.

If they could spend less time in the courtroom and more time in the research lab, maybe they could perfect a way to get fetuses hooked in utero (can this be?) or better yet, create fads for kids to associate smoking with fun (like Smokémon instead of Pokémon trading cards).

Your friend, PJ ✚

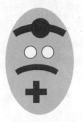

Why Couldn't You Hate Me?

One of my chronic pain patients who I have been shepherding along for years with many peaks and valleys came to see me. She was very depressed. It was the holiday season and she had to see her mother *(and she hates her mother).* This patient was also having severe sleep difficulties (prolonged latency and early morning awakening) despite Elavil 150 mg and Klonopin 2 mg for restless legs.

"Why are you telling this to me? I'm your pain doctor. You have a psychiatrist, a neurologist, and a psychologist."

"Yes, but you're my favorite."

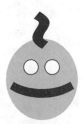

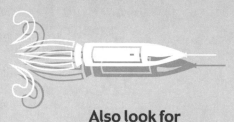
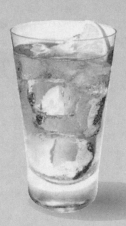

X-Ray Files

If we show you ours, will you show us yours?

Adding ears to an MRI scan
is nothing to scrunch your nose at.

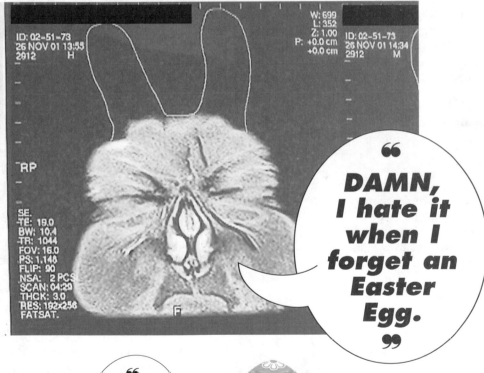

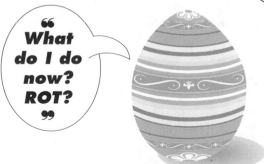

Medical Brush

A few years ago I read a newspaper story about an upcoming visit to Our Fair City by none other than **John Wayne Bobbitt.**

I have been a big fan of amputee sex stories ever since the *Penthouse* Letters I read back in the 70s, so I knew I HAD to see this show, which was playing at a local topless bar. I tried to get together a gang of my medical colleagues to go see Bobbitt. Unfortunately nobody would go, except my friend Bill, a urologist. Most doctors are afraid to go to these establishments. Not because it's unprofessional, but because they are scared they may be spotted by patients (*both the patrons and dancers*).

I didn't give a sh#t. This was John Wayne Bobbitt for God's sake!

When Bill's wife heard about the planned trip, she tried to keep him from going. I subsequently threatened Bill that if he backed out I'd let everybody know he was "whipped." So we set out on a sunny Saturday afternoon. After paying the cover charge (*interesting term for a place where not being covered is the main attraction*) we entered into the main room, where we got some cheap steak-like substances from the buffet and sat down to wait for the show.

We ordered drinks and turned down a couple of overtures from some Ladies of Negotiable Affection. Then the lights dimmed. The spotlights came on. The emcee announced the "man we have all been waiting for," and then there he was, "John . . . Wayne . . . Bobbitt!" In a tuxedo!

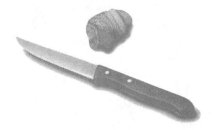

John told maybe three insipid jokes and then showed a tape from the Howard Stern Show re-enacting the Big Event. After that, the "Bobbitt Girls" came out and waggled their bobbitts at us. There was enough silicone there to caulk all the pools in Florida. After the show

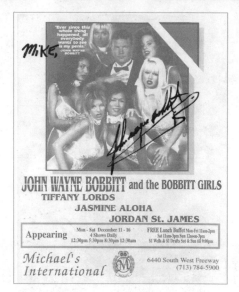

Mike,

"Ever since this whole thing happened, all everybody wants to see is my penis."
—JOHN WAYNE BOBBITT

JOHN WAYNE BOBBITT and the **BOBBITT GIRLS**
TIFFANY LORDS
JASMINE ALOHA
JORDAN St. JAMES

Appearing | Mon - Sat December 11 - 16 | FREE Lunch Buffet Mon-Fri 11am-2pm
4 Shows Daily | Sat 11am-3pm Sun 12noon-3pm
12:30pm 5:30pm 8:30pm 12:30am | $1 Wells & $3 Drafts Sat & Sun till 9:00pm

Michael's International 6440 South West Freeway
(713) 784-5900

John and his Girls were available for autographs. We got him to sign one for each of us (above). Then we mentioned that we were "trained medical doctors" and had a "professional interest in seeing his medical miracle."

We could have been anybody wanting to look at his private parts but for some reason, John trusted us. *Maybe it was the sincere way we managed to keep a straight face.* We persuaded John to go into the men's room with us so we could inspect his "object of interest." There we were: Bill the urologist, John Wayne Bobbitt, and me in the men's room, with John whipping out one of the most famous phalluses this country has ever known. It was a sight to see. We knew we were breaking the ancient "Never Look at Another Guy in the Men's Room Especially Below the Waist" rule but we ignored it as well as the curious sidelong glances from the other denizens taking a bladder break. Bill and I felt since this was the opportunity of a lifetime for a physician – to hell with rules.

As I stated, Bill is a urologist and I guess he is used to seeing these things up close. This is probably why he stuck his face right into John Wayne Bobbitt's crotch to get a better look (*much closer than necessary in my humble opinion*).

"It looks like you've had some fat injected there to give it support," said Bill, who truly seemed fascinated and wouldn't stop staring.

with Greatness

"Ever since this whole thing happened, all everybody wants to see is my penis."

John Wayne Bobbitt

"Never mind that," I said, breaking Bill's trance, *"Mr. Bobbitt, I have a huge favor to ask you."* I pulled an ink pad from my back pocket. *"Would you mind making an imprint for us as a souvenir?"*

From what I had seen of John on TV and just witnessed up close and personal, I knew that he wasn't a mental genius. Still, I was surprised at his reply. *"Is that stuff safe?"* he asked me.

"Mr. Bobbitt," I assured him, *"as we explained before, we are trained medical doctors. This ink pad is the very same kind that we use to make baby footprints for birth certificates. Surely if it's safe enough for a newborn baby it's safe enough for you."*

With these ridiculous and totally unverifiable assurances, John walked over to the sink, put the pad on the counter and smooshed his "famous member" into the ink and then onto a piece of paper (right). Twice; one for me and one for Bill.

We thanked John profusely and started to leave with our trophies, trying not to rupture our tracheas with suppressed laughter.

"Are you sure this stuff will come off?" he called after us.

To which I replied over my shoulder, *"Absolutely – just use a little alcohol. Vodka will do nicely. Ask the bartender."*

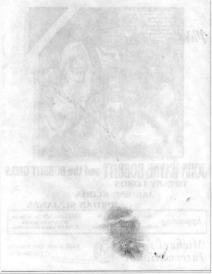

And with that, Bill and I walked out giving each other high fives. It was like two kids getting Barry Bond's autograph. I said we were medical professionals but I didn't say we were mature medical professionals.

I later found that my Bobbitt-grams were in big demand, so I made photocopies and handed them out. I discovered this interesting fact about human nature: people will not touch a photocopy of an imprint of a man's penis. Even when I reminded them that it was a photocopy, and not the original, people still wouldn't touch it. Some wouldn't even hold the paper in their hands. For grins, sometimes I'd hand them to people and ask them to guess what it was. They'd study it carefully and usually give up. When I told them what they were holding they went through a bobbling routine like Curly from the Three Stooges, except most of them didn't go "Woo woo woo woo! Hey Larry! Hey Moe!"

Some of you are probably wondering if I still have the ink pad. I don't. Although I was tempted to use it to stamp "Past Due" on delinquent patient bills, on the way to the parking lot I threw it in the trash. I bought my secretary a replacement the following Monday. ✚

GET OFF THE ROAD

A few years ago, I was telling a patient with chronic schizophrenia about a new antipsychotic med I was prescribing for her. I mentioned that it could make her drowsy and she should be very careful not to drive or "operate any machinery."

Her eyes widened suddenly and she asked *"Can I still use a vibrator?"*

(I answered *"Yes"* and suppressed a desire to quip, *"Yes, just not while driving."*) ✚

is *it* in you?

Joe presented to the ER with a Gatorade bottle stuck in his rectum. Having been there for quite a while it had caused some bowel damage which necessitated a surgery for removal of the bottle and a temporary colostomy.

When the recovery nurses were taking the patient to his room, the television was on. While they were moving him from the gurney to the bed, the Gatorade commercial came on saying, **"Gatorade - is *it* in you?"** The nurses cracked up and had to leave the room.

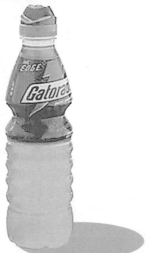

One afternoon, I joked around thinking a certain patient was out of earshot; she was not. She asked my nurse a question, *"Will this new medication interact with any of my current medications?"* I replied,

"Yes, it will result in a painful seizure that will last about an hour before she dies . . ."

It was only after these words were spoken that she leaned around the door to let me know that she had heard this comment. Not surprisingly, that was the first and last time I ever saw her. ✚

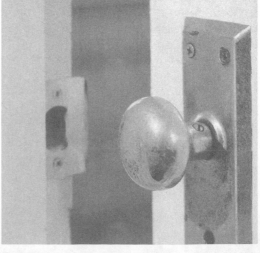

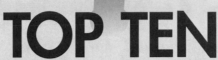

TOP TEN
Ways Physicians Piss Off Drug Reps

10 Forgets who you are even though she has seen you over 400 times.

9 Invites everyone he knows to a dine and dash (pre-PhRMA* days) including his staff, his neighbors, other people in the restaurant, and even the guy who carries the sign *"Wil Wurk For Food."*

8 Promises that she has been using tons of your drug even though the numbers state she has never written even one prescription.

7 Hides when you walk into the office and won't come out of his room until you leave (*which you won't*).

6 Pretends you are invisible to the point of almost walking through you.

5 Shows up at the very last minute to your lunch after you have fed his whole staff and then becomes indignant when you want to even mention the name of your drug.

4 She never speaks to you, yet claims a national emergency if her samples are out and demands you come refill it (*even then she still won't speak to you*).

3 Pretends to be a celebrity by not letting you see him, but instead has his nurse carry the signature pad to him making you feel like a groupie getting an autograph.

2 Comes to your lecture at a local restaurant late and either falls asleep, talks to his friend, or leaves right after the main course (*taking his dessert home in a doggie bag*).

1 He actually spends time with you, but uses it to berate you, your company, and prescription drugs in general.

---

* Pharmaceutical Research and Manufacturers of America, a lobbyist group for the pharmaceutical industry

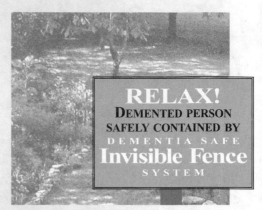

HUNG-RY LIKE THE WOLF

They say if his nose is wet, he's healthy.

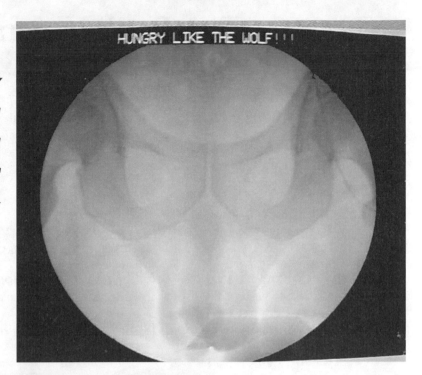

X-Ray Files

FUN WITH TV CHARACTERS

COOKIE MONSTER? ▶
What are you doing on that scrotal ultrasound!

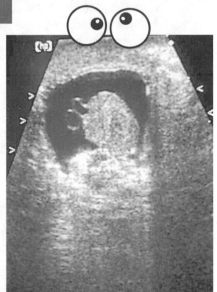

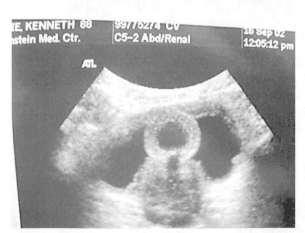

◀ **IS IT KENNY?**

He's not dead, he's in this bladder ultrasound!

Things I STILL Don't Understand After Being in the ED for 15 Years

The Famous "While I'm" Visit. You cannot figure out why this patient is here with her problem until she says, *"I was visiting my mother upstairs in room 342, and I thought that while I'm here, I thought I would be seen."*

The teenage imperative to wear a baseball cap while being otherwise undressed for an exam.

The "Party of Five" visit. Suddenly in the middle of the busiest Sunday of the year, the triage nurse dumps five charts on the desk. You go to examine this group, thinking that Mom has brought in all five kids, and find out that **three of them are not hers!** They are nieces' or neighbors' kids! *What do people do before they leave for the ED?* Do they call around the neighborhood and ask if anybody needs anything while she is going out? *"Yeah,"* replies a friend. *"Can you take little Mike to the ED and get him seen for this cough?"*

The patient with the sick kid who has an appointment with their pediatrician in twenty minutes, who came to the ED because they *"couldn't wait that long"* to see their own doctor.

Why do patients think that their child with the nausea and vomiting should undergo the Doritos Challenge in the ED?

And why do patients think that their Primary Care MD is going to meet them in the ED at 9 p.m.? Probably for the same reason that they ask you why the subspecialist that they need is not in residence at the hospital at 1:32 a.m.

I never understand the patient who queries my nurse, *"Do I have to undress?"* No you idiot, the doctor has X-ray vision!

"My child just isn't herself." (Who the hell is she?) Enough said.

"To tell you the truth Doc . . ." What? Have you been lying up to this point?

"I hate to go to doctors." Why the hell did you have to have a change of heart tonight!

"I've had this problem *for two years, and neither my primary nor the three specialists she had me see can tell me what it is. Can you diagnose it?"* **Yeah, right!!!**

Why do patients think it's okay to eat pizza, subs and burgers in the exam room?

And my favorite. It always appears to come from some baseball cap–wearing, pimply-faced 16-year-old . . . You introduce yourself to the patient and get a dead mackerel handshake. You ask the patient what is wrong and they reply . . .

"I don't know, you're the doctor!"

A real Henny Youngman!!!! ✚

180

STRATEGIC FILIBUSTERING
AT YOUR NEXT
HOSPITAL COMMITTEE MEETING

1. Ask for more data – this always works. Use phrases like "level of confidence is low" or "statistically insignificant" to scare the members into searching for more data. This data is never available.

2. Ask for whatever data you have to be "analyzed" in a more effective manner – use phrases like "confounding variables" or "background noise" to make the members skeptical.

3. Ask for more members to be added to the group – everyone knows that more is better, but since everyone hates committees, you'll never get anyone to join.

4. Ask to have a consultant brought in – somehow this fools even the best of them. You have to first debate if a consultant is needed, and then debate what type of consultant to get. Even if you get an answer on this, you still have to find a way to pay the consultant. There is never money in the budget to pay a consultant.

5. Ask to have the group broken down into smaller task forces, steering committees or action groups – by the time you define what the goal of the "microcommittee" is, you will head right into the realization that no one will volunteer to be on it.

6. Ask to bring the issue to the largest group of the hospital (general staff meeting, etc.) – by the law of averages, some crotchety bastard will hate the issue enough to force it back into the smaller committee again where you can filibuster it all over again.

7. Try bringing up a point and then slowly, but deliberately go tangential – by the time the committee realizes you are on another topic, you make sure that new topic is really controversial. That will piss off your "hothead" in the group enough to have him speak his mind about the new topic and you are now off to the races. Sit back and enjoy.

8. Ask to have a consensus on the issue and then try to have the committee define *consensus* and see if they can have a consensus on that definition.

9. Ask your "slowspeaker" in the group to give their in-depth opinion and when she does, ask her more questions on how she can elaborate on what she just said.

10. Ask if the issue at hand is really that important when so many other issues are critical (they never are) – try to table this issue and promise to bring it up on the next meeting and then reapply any one of the top nine techniques. ✚

TOP TEN

Things I've Always Wanted to Say to Patients
(but luckily never came out of my mouth!)

10 "I think that your toilet is developing a Lortab addiction."

9 "So it hurts when you carry something that weighs 150 lbs . . . Don't do that, God didn't include that in your warranty."

8 "It is my policy to not biopsy something that cannot be detected by my five senses, a CT, MRI and $3,100 of blood work, or any of the six specialists you've seen . . ."

7 "I'm willing to talk to you about anything today except what you have been doing in the bathroom for the past week."

6 "I'm not getting rich giving flu shots, so don't consider that you are doing me a personal favor if you take one . . ."

5 "There is nothing wrong with you below the neck . . ."

4 "Would you consider having a tubal ligation/vasectomy . . . at my expense?"

3 "Will Rogers couldn't have been your doctor . . ."

2 "I'm a lot sicker than you are today and you don't see me asking for a work excuse . . ."

1 (acting surprised) "We haven't MRI'd that (fill in the blank) this month?" ✚

AFTER 30 YEARS AS AN ER DOC:
MY FAVORITE TRUE STORIES OF MEDICINE

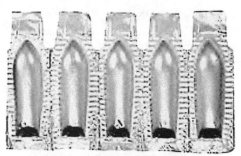

A patient complaining of constipation still had the suppositories recommended by the doctor in his rectum – *with the tin foil still on them.*

A mother who was told to go to the Ped Clinic the next day for follow-up did indeed show up, *but left the baby at home.*

A mother put amoxicillin into the baby's ears for an ear infection. *(It should be swallowed.)*

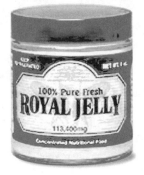

A man came in with a jar of King Kelly's Royal Jelly in his rectum. He said that he fell asleep at a party and when he awoke, wouldn't you know it, there it was. After a rather difficult extraction, he came back two weeks later with the same problem. *I've got a feeling he may be lying or he needs a better circle of friends.*

A man put a large nut onto his penis in order to maintain an erection but he could not get it off. Since it was of tempered steel, the fire department had to be called in order to cut the thing. The carbon steel saw generated so much heat, the nurse had to continually pour water over the area so that the patient's penis would not get burned. *OUCH!* +

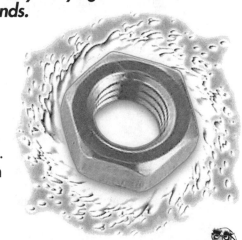

I am a registered nurse, and I love reading each issue of *Placebo Journal*. However, I am also a PHARMACEUTICAL REP and I've had just about enough of your insulting, critical comments regarding my line of work! So, I thought I'd let you and your readers know what it's REALLY like to be a drug rep. I'll call my piece ...

I know doctors are very busy and I really try to respect their time(honestly) while simultaneously fulfilling my job requirements. I try to have some pertinent piece of information to share as quickly as possible. I try to be pleasant, brief, and helpful. Mercifully, some of my docs respond well to this tactic. Following is a sampling of some of the physicians that make my job so much fun ... see if you recognize yourself:

DR. FIBBS Upon seeing me in his office, immediately he begins declaring, *"I use your drug a lot. I know all about it."* When, in fact, the lying bastard doesn't use it at all. Just give it to me straight, Doc. I'd prefer a brusque *"I hate your drug. Don't come back to me, okay?"* over a lie any day. But I realize this is just a technique to send us on our way without wasting more time than necessary. That is why I can't be too angry with Dr. Fibbs.

DR. LUNCHESONLY He's elusive and mysterious (but not in a good way). Sometimes, when I bring lunch into one of these offices, some staffer will have pity on me and actually say something to me like, *"Thanks for lunch"* while grabbing her food and bolting for the door. *(Oops! Don't forget to take a lunch to your boyfriend/ husband/ child waiting around the corner!)* If I'm lucky, the doctor may make an appearance, like a surprise celebrity guest on a talk show. *Does he use my drug at least?* Who knows? (That's the mysterious part.)

DR. FLIRTY EYES I call on about 250 physicians, and Dr. Flirty Eyes is the only one who turns me into a demure babbling idiot who speaks intelligibly. *"I am a professional,"* I tell myself. *"Just go in there and avoid eye contact. Just give your detail and get the hell out before he looks at you with his flirty eyes!"* Dr. Flirty Eyes does something to me, alright. If only he'd just ignore me like so many other doctors. Problem is, he is one if my most "important" customers, so I have to see him on a regular basis. Okay, okay. So I'm human. *It's not like I'm sleeping with him.* Or dreaming about it . . . *hmmm.*

DR. CODGER hates everything, everyone, himself, the world, etc. Every time I see him, he lectures me on how the world is going to hell because of pharmaceutical companies, Medicare, the government, and immoral people in general. Last time, he spewed on and on about the moral decline of today's youth and how no one takes marriage seriously any more. (This caused sharp guilt pangs, considering my feelings for Dr. Flirty Eyes.) Generally, I like this type of doctor, though. They seem to need someone to "vent" to, and after all, *I am there to take care of my customers.*

MORE THAN A PEN WHORE

DR. RANDY I call on Dr. Randy because I know his staff won't get miffed if I use their bathroom when it has been seven hours since I last voided and my bladder is about to burst. Last time I went to Dr. Randy's office, I looked like a drowned rat (having been out and about in the rain all day). My hair was frizzy, my makeup was streaked, my clothes were wet, and I smelled like the fast food I had scarfed for lunch. I got soaked walking into the office *(I always park away from the building so as not to take the prime spots from patients – TRUE)*, and I was told to wait. I knew I'd get in to see him because he tells everyone to let in the "hot ones" *(TRUE)* and apparently, I'm hot *(debatable)*. Although on this particular day I looked like a drowned rat, as I mentioned earlier, so *ha ha!* The joke was on him! But alas, the joke was on me. Dr. Randy just stared at my breasts during the whole visit. *What was there to see except a bulky raincoat?* I don't worry about what he thinks when I laugh out loud at him. He probably thinks I'm a bimbo anyway and a giggling, bouncing chest just adds to the charm, *right?*

DR. NEWBIE Meeting doctors who are new in town is usually a challenge because I have to prove to them that I'm not a twenty-three year-old with a business degree who knows nothing about patient care. The younger ones respect my clinical background. The older ones just think I'm a low-life nurse who only knows how to take orders. How infuriating to be ignored, while the males reps are taken seriously! Poor me *(sigh)*. *Maybe I should take off the raincoat?* Just kidding. *Puh-lease.* As if.

DR. SERIOUS He and others like him worry me the most. I honestly believe that this man has never smiled a day in his life. Dr. Serious is very serious about his patients, about life, about medications, about the weather. He happened to be standing in line behind me one day at a local restaurant. We were each there with some friends. I caught his eye, smiled, and said *"Hello,"* and then went back to thinking about how miserably full I was. Just then, he put up his hand – crossing-guard style – and proclaimed (loudly), *"No offense, but I don't talk to reps outside of my office. My personal life is my personal life!"* Okaaaayyyy. Next time I'm out in public, Doc, I'll make sure to go incognito so you won't be bothered. *Sheesh!* Just because some of your drug reps are overbearing leeches, doesn't mean that I am. Besides, I have a life, too, you know. Why do you think I'm peddling pharmaceuticals? I got tired of working 16-hour shifts, and on nights, weekends, and holidays in a grueling job that doesn't pay enough. *Sound familiar?* You're not the only ones with families! *Besides, I look sexy in the company minivan.*

DR. BALANCED He is rare indeed. He laughs, smiles, cares about his patients, and is courteous to everyone, including the evil souls who represent pharmaceutical companies. His patients and staff love him. He finds time to play golf. I look at the many pictures of his family placed all around his office. I wonder how he does it. *How does he manage to stay so happy within the confines of the modern medical system?* It must be Valium, I think. Then I spy the most recent issue of *Placebo Journal* on his desk. ✚

P.S. *If one more f%*ker asks for a f*#king pen . . .*

GUNPOINT B#OWJOB

This is a true story. I have not altered nor enhanced the story one word.

I am an ER physician working in a small community hospital in northwest Florida. I was working the 7 p.m. to 7 a.m. shift. I had discharged the last patient at 3 a.m. and headed for the call room. I lay down and dearly hoped that I would get some sleep. Two hours later, at 5 a.m., I got a call that we had a new patient. I went into Room #5 to see a young man perched on the edge of the bed, sitting bolt upright. He was rubbing his hands together nervously when I walked in.

"Hi, I'm Dr. ————. Tell me what brings you in tonight."

"Well," he replied anxiously, clearly searching for words, *"I guess you would say that I was sexually assaulted."*

I looked at this robust 27-year-old guy, who appeared to be about 6'2", probably 220 pounds; broad shoulders, not an ounce of fat on him, and thought to myself, *"Who could have overpowered this guy?"* As unbelievable as his story sounded, I still had to play the role of compassionate physician.

"Oh, I'm terribly sorry. I can only imagine how upsetting that must be. What exactly happened?"

Slowly he began, *"I had been at the bar last night. I guess I left around 3 a.m. Driving home I saw a woman hitchhiking. Since it was cold out, I felt sorry for her and picked her up. I offered to drive her home and she began giving me directions. Turn left* here, turn right there, and so on. Next thing I knew, we were in a pretty desolate location, and it was pitch dark.

"She then said, 'Well, I guess you know what time it is.'

"What do you mean?" I asked.

"Then she pulled out a gun, pointed it at me and said, 'Give me all your sh#t!'

"Realizing that I was being robbed, I reached into my back pocket and gave her my wallet.

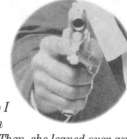

'You've got something else I want,' she said. 'Pull your pants down.'

"I was scared, but hey, she had a gun! So I pulled my pants down halfway to my knees. Then, she leaned over and 'went down' on me."

"She gave you oral sex?"

I asked incredulously, "Right there in the car . . . at GUNPOINT?"

"Yeah."

Having trouble picturing this I asked, "How long did this go on?"

He hesitated, "Uh-h-h, 5, 10, 15 minutes."

"What happened next?" I asked.

"She got out of the car, ordered me not to tell anyone, and ran into the darkness."

You hear all kinds of crazy things in the ER, but I never heard a story like that. "You've called the police, of course." I asked.

"Oh, no!" he replied, suddenly getting more nervous.

"Why not?"

"Uh-h-h-h, there's nothing for them to do. I mean, it's over and done. They can't do anything now."

I responded by saying, "Look, the law requires me to call the police anytime I see a victim of violence or assault here in the ER. I will have to call the police. Besides, doesn't she have your wallet, your driver's license, and your credit cards?"

He thought about it a minute then said, "No. She went through my wallet, took out the only money I had – about five dollars – then gave the wallet back to me."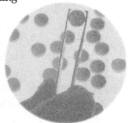

This story was getting more ridiculous by the moment. Finally, I said, "Well, if you don't want to talk to the police, and if you were not injured, why did you come here? What do you want me to do for you?"

Then came the "answer."

"I'm afraid I might have caught something. You know, an STD. So I want some kind of shot or a pill . . . so that I won't catch anything. When she went down on me she kinda chewed on me . . . kinda bit me a couple of times . . . I-I-I don't want to catch anything."

Oh-h-h!! Now I get it!! Now I understand!!

This idiot paid some hooker for oral sex. Then, when the deed was done, he suddenly regained his senses and thought, "Uh-oh! I've done a bad thing!" Now he wants a "magic shot" to make it all go away.

One of my moral impurities is that of a great sense of humor. I was tempted to say to him, "Hey, count yourself lucky!! A strange woman gives you oral sex on your way home from the bar, only charges you five bucks plus a ride

home, and you HAD to sit still for it because she was holding a GUN on you!! You can tell your wife, or girlfriend, (or both), that you had NO choice in the matter and that NONE of this was your fault. You HAD to go along with it because 'your life was in jeopardy!!' And of course, you couldn't disarm her even though she is sitting right next to you in the confined space of a car, FACEDOWN, WITH HER HEAD BURIED IN YOUR LAP. Oh, no. There was NO WAY to disarm her. Heck, I doubt if even Rambo or Bruce Lee could have gotten out of THAT 'life-threatening' situation!!" Despite the temptation, I kept my thoughts to myself.

Of course, as the doctor, I was obligated to perform an exam. His genitals were uninjured except for a slight red mark of the side of the penile shaft. The mark's length and width were consistent with that of a front incisor tooth. No skin was broken anywhere, no bruising, no other evidence of trauma, etc.

I explained that the likelihood of contracting an STD from oral sex was low. If he developed any symptoms of syphilis, gonorrhea, or chlamydia, he should return for treatment. To my knowledge, there have been no documented cases of seroconversion for HIV by oral sex. Furthermore, if he caught herpes, HPV, or hepatitis, there wasn't a whole lot to be done anyway. So the best thing for him to do was just lick his wounds (*pun intended*), hope he didn't catch anything, and learn from his mistakes.

My cruel sense of humor tempted me to offer this idiot emergency contraception . . . you know, the "morning after pill," but I didn't think the hospital pharmacy would dispense it to a male.

Finally, as I was walking out of the exam room, I was tempted to ask, "By the way, exactly where did yo drop her off?" After all, my shift ends in two hours.

✚

MY FAVORITE MUNCHAUSEN

SHE'S NO COLORING BOOK

Leslie was a young girl with an affinity for making accusations. Her stories were many, but most of the time they included being sexually assaulted. In this instance, Leslie made things worse by refusing to be medically examined. This is where our physician hero comes in. He was a good doc and extremely thorough as Leslie's charges were serious. This is where our story begins.

Leslie claimed to be 15 years old but looked suspiciously older. She stated that she was raped, bitten, punched, and pilfered (amongst other things). No one initially doubted our lady, as no one should with these kind of accusations. Unfortunately, Leslie's story didn't seem quite right. Her arms showed track lines consistent with drug use, but Leslie denied them all. She did have small lacerations, but they were what our doctor called a "self-harm" pattern. Her bite marks were similar to forcible pinching, probably done by Leslie herself. *Hmmm.* The rest of the exam became more and more difficult as Leslie stopped cooperating. Even when the doctor noticed "colored objects" in her vaginal area, Leslie would play no part in this charade and wanted out.

Eventually, the rest of the examination was forcibly done under anesthesia because the seriousness of the charges demanded a full report. Sure, it may seem weird that the colored objects that the physician first saw turned out to be NINE CRAYONS. Unfortunately, our little Munchausen didn't stop there.

Twelve hours after the anesthesia was given, Leslie seemed to have had grand-mal seizures that developed into a status epilepticus-like condition. *This could have been life threatening!* She needed an intensive care transfer and intubation. After being on the ventilator overnight, Leslie's blood was found to contain morphine and tranquilizers. This is when our physician got more curious.

Luckily, the police were very helpful in this case. A search showed that Leslie had made many similar complaints around the country, most of which included being sexually assaulted and most of which included crayons. *Where was this crayon bandit?* Only Leslie knew and he must have been following her around.

Leslie was eventually found to be 24 years old with tons of aliases. During other hospitalizations, she was found to have bad seizures also and they were caused by taking overdoses in the hospital. Sometimes she would cut herself to stay longer. Whatever it took, Leslie would do.

Like a typical Munchausen, Leslie denied the charges when confronted. She left the hospital against medical advice and did not take the crayons. When asked by the police where she was going, Leslie responded, *"I'm off to the next big city."*

The story wasn't over. Our physician noticed that four months later Leslie was admitted to another hospital and received a laparoscopy for abdominal pain after being "sexually assaulted" again. This time a metal bottle top and clear glass was found within her vagina. Still not over. A few days later she was admitted to another hospital in a different county claiming her laparoscopy scars were due to being stabbed in the stomach by a person sexually assaulting her.

The whereabouts of Leslie are now unknown. The police are still looking for her because of theft and fraud charges. Therefore, if you find a patient with interesting objects inserted "down under" who can fake a seizure like nobody's business, we at *Placebo Journal* recommend you give them a call. ✚

This story was liberally embellished from:
Med. Sci. Law *(1998), Vol. 38, No. 3*

CONCLUSION

So that is it. You finished *The Placebo Chronicles*, which may be your first medical book. *Okay, maybe you can't define this as a true medical book from a purist's perspective.* Skeptics may point to the fact that real medical books are at least informative and educational. My response to them is that those same books are boring, tedious, and long-winded. Sure you didn't learn crap about practicing medicine from *The Placebo Chronicles* but will those other books ever make one of their readers incontinent because they laughed so hard?

In reality, your journey through *The Placebo Chronicles* was small glimpses through many different physicians' lives. This book wasn't one story unto itself and that makes it difficult to bring it to a neat conclusion. I could try to end it like my old teachers used to do in medical school. They had a standard technique for finishing each class. First, they would sum up the all the important points they just lectured about. Second, they would reinforce how much we, as students, needed to know those points. Lastly, they would test us at a later date on something totally different from what they taught. It was their way of saying, *"Screw you for sleeping through my class."* Or maybe that was just the way I perceived it.

Obviously I don't want you to feel the way those teachers made me feel. What I can do is thank you for your interest. We physicians are caretakers and as caretakers it is nice to see that those we take care of have some interest in our lives as well. I hope that the material in *The Placebo Chronicles* either made you laugh, smile, or in some way piqued your interest. I will still deem this book a success, however, if you are now able to empathize with the doctors you just read about. *And if I make money from it.* I hope that by living through their embarrassment, their pain, and their humor you can conclude that doctors are human with all the weaknesses inherent to everyone. We pretend to be creatures of logic, but in reality we are creatures of emotion (humor, sympathy, depression, and anger) just like everyone else. Ignoring this concept, which unfortunately many doctors around the world still do, only causes us more problems in the long run. Welcoming these emotions enables doctors to be better people, be better at their job, or to be at least somewhat sociable at the next party.

Before you leave this book next to the toilet, I ask that you do a couple of things. First, for God's sake, wash your hands. Second, try not to judge poorly any of the physicians who have written some of these stories. I know I try not to. I feel that until I walk in another doctor's moccasins, get another person's cavity fluid splashed in my mouth, or find some fresh infant stool left in my office trash can, I will continue to reserve any judgment on another doctor. I hope you can do the same; the judgment part, I mean, and not the cavity-fluid-in-mouth thing.

Lastly, I want to warn you about the future. The media, the politicians, and the cynics will always try to convince us that medicine is in crisis. I am going to let you in on a little secret: **medicine has always been in crisis.** Even in the Middle Ages when they were using leeches, some administrators were trying to save money by allowing only generic bloodletting. The only thing holding steadfast throughout time is that physicians have always been there to help people. Because of this, the medical system will survive and maybe more importantly, *The Placebo Chronicles* will have more stories to share with you in the future. ✚

ACKNOWLEDGMENTS

I have so many people to thank for helping get this book together. *The Placebo Chronicles* is a consortium of not only stories but the people who helped make them happen. Just because my name is on the cover doesn't mean that they shouldn't be recognized or paid. Since there is no way I will be doing the latter, I will try and make it up here. Hopefully that will get them off my back.

I want to thank my wife, Debbie, who has always been there by my side and has talked me out of quitting on multiple occasions. She has put up with more of my "projects" than any wife should have to. She never really believed that I was a real doctor. Now with the publication of *The Placebo Chronicles* she is probably going to feel justified.

I want to thank Gordon Marshall. He is the best graphic design artist and illustrator a rookie magazine publisher could ever have. I told you when we started that we would make it someday. Please don't leave me now that you are big and famous.

I want to thank my literary agent, Bob Mecoy, who felt even a family doctor could make it as a writer. The bigger question is can a writer make it as a family doctor? He hung on and pushed for a deal even when the going was tough. Promising the whole Broadway Books division that I would provide all their medical care was probably not appropriate, however.

I want to thank Reneé Catacalos. As a long-time friend and confident, she helped me market the *Placebo Journal* for only a small pittance. She is not only a public relations genius but also grammatical expert as well. Without her, my thoughts would not convert to paper nearly as well. I usually no write so good. See, I could have used you right there, Reneé.

I want to thank Charlie Conrad at Broadway Books for giving me a chance. I hope our relationship in this business continues for a long time. I could use the money. Being a family physician doesn't pay like it used to.

I want to thank Dr. Michael Gorback for his insane opinions and great stories. I never thought any other physician could be as weird as I am. I was wrong.

I especially want to thank Dr. Susan Summerton and Dr. Joe Ullman for contributing many of the X-rays and stories for this book. It is awesome to see radiologists with such a great sense of humor. Actually it is nice to see a radiologist with any sense of humor.

I want to thank my medical partners at Court Street Family Practice. Drs. Ray Stone, Carolyn Kase, and John Comis are not only great physicians but wonderful friends. Without your support I would have quit medicine or jumped in front of a moving train a long time ago.

I want to thank my kids. Jake, Lucas, and Niki are the true treasures of my life. Thank you for understanding the times I wasn't with you and for being quiet when "Daddy is working in his office." Also, I want to thank you years ahead of time for not spending all my money on tuition, cars, or indiscretionary purchases.

Lastly, I want to thank all the doctors, too many to name, who have contributed stories to both the *Placebo Journal* and *The Placebo Chronicles.* This book will hopefully show to the world that doctors are human too. It will also be something for you to show your loved ones who thought you were uptight, humorless, and stressed out. ✚

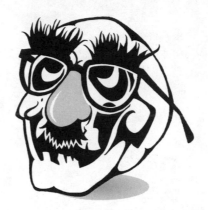

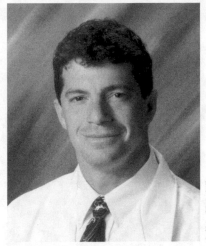
© Skip Churchill

ABOUT THE AUTHOR

Douglas Farrago, M.D., is a family physician who started the bimonthly *Placebo Journal* in 2000. A frequent lecturer and media commentator, Dr. Farrago lives in Auburn, Maine.